100 Questions & Answers About Hysterectomy

Delthia Ricks, MA, MS
Medical Writer
Newsday
Long Island, New York

Lloyd B. Greig, MD
Department of Obstetrics and Gynecology
The Cedars Sinai Medical Group
Beverly Hills, California

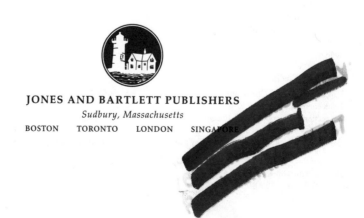

JONES AND BARTLETT PUBLISHERS
Sudbury, Massachusetts
BOSTON   TORONTO   LONDON   SINGAPORE

World Headquarters
Jones and Bartlett Publishers
40 Tall Pine Drive
Sudbury, MA 01776
978-443-5000
info@jbpub.com
www.jbpub.com

Jones and Bartlett Publishers
Canada
6339 Ormindale Way
Mississauga, Ontario
L5V 1J2
CANADA

Jones and Bartlett Publishers
International
Barb House, Barb Mews
London W6 7PA
UK

Jones and Bartlett's books and products are available through most bookstores and online booksellers. To contact Jones and Bartlett Publishers directly, call 800-832-0034, fax 978-443-8000, or visit our website www.jbpub.com.

Substantial discounts on bulk quantities of Jones and Bartlett's publications are available to corporations, professional associations, and other qualified organizations. For details and specific discount information, contact the special sales department at Jones and Bartlett via the above contact information or send an email to specialsales@jbpub.com.

The authors, editor, and publisher have made every effort to provide accurate information. However, they are not responsible for errors, omissions, or for any outcomes related to the use of the contents of this book and take no responsibility for the use of the products described. Treatments and side effects described in this book may not be applicable to all patients; likewise, some patients may require a dose or experience a side effect that is not described herein. The reader should confer with his or her own physician regarding specific treatments and side effects. Drugs and medical devices are discussed that may have limited availability controlled by the Food and Drug Administration (FDA) for use only in a research study or clinical trial. The drug information presented has been derived from reference sources, recently published data, and pharmaceutical research data. Research, clinical practice, and government regulations often change the accepted standard in this field. When consideration is being given to use of any drug in the clinical setting, the health care provider or reader is responsible for determining FDA status of the drug, reading the package insert, reviewing prescribing information for the most up-to-date recommendations on dose, precautions, and contraindications, and determining the appropriate usage for the product. This is especially important in the case of drugs that are new or seldom used.

Library of Congress Cataloging-in-Publication Data

Ricks, Delthia.
100 questions & answers about hysterectomy / Delthia Ricks, Lloyd B. Greig.
   p. cm.
Includes index.
ISBN-13: 978-0-7637-3463-3 (alk. paper)
ISBN-10: 0-7637-3463-2 (alk. paper)
   1. Hysterectomy--Miscellanea. I. Greig, Lloyd B. II. Title. III. Title: One hundred questions and answers about hysterectomy.
RG391.R52 2007
618.1'453--dc22
        2006017083

6048

Production Credits

Executive Publisher: Christopher Davis
Production Director: Amy Rose
Production Editor: Carolyn F. Rogers
Associate Editor: Kathy Richardson
Associate Marketing Manager: Laura Kavigian

Manufacturing Buyer: Therese Connell
Composition: Jason Miranda, Spoke & Wheel
Cover Design: Kate Ternullo
Printing and Binding: Malloy, Inc.
Cover Printing: Malloy, Inc.

Printed in the United States of America
10 09 08 07 06   10 9 8 7 6 5 4 3 2 1

Contents

I have to say with all honesty that even though I was diagnosed with fibroids, I didn't know that I had them, at least not at first. They apparently had been developing for many years, maybe as long as a decade but probably much longer. I was in my late forties when they were first brought to my attention. If I hadn't gone in for my annual pelvic exam, which is when the doctor discovered them, I probably would have been unaware for a lot longer. He told me at the time: "If they aren't bothering you, leave them alone. There's no need for surgery or any other procedure if you're not experiencing symptoms."

I am a registered nurse and I am well aware of symptoms—what to suspect, what to look for. But regarding the issue of fibroids, I wasn't connecting the doctor's diagnosis to one of my major symptoms, which in this case was urinary frequency. I had always had urinary frequency, but for some reason I just didn't attribute it to the fibroids. For one thing, I had experienced urinary frequency from the time I was in elementary school. So it was nothing new to me. My children were aware of the problem, too. They would say: "Oh no, Mom's got to go [to the bathroom], get out of the way." The need to urinate would occur so suddenly and with such urgency that I was always making a beeline to the bathroom.

And I must admit that prior to my hysterectomy there were times when urinary frequency could be embarrassing. I remember being incontinent on occasion; the urine would flow uncontrollably, no matter where I was. I learned very quickly how to avoid this, especially when I was in public places. When I went out I wouldn't drink excessive amounts of fluid. I knew that if I drank water, I would have to run immediately to the bathroom. For some reason that wasn't the case with coffee even though I was well aware, at least from what I had read, that coffee can act as a diuretic. For me it never was, and I drink coffee frequently. My biggest fear, the thing I was most apprehensive about, was an eight-ounce glass of water because that would always pass straight through and I would have to run to the nearest bathroom.

As the years passed, and the fibroids progressed there was another symptom—a textbook symptom to tell the truth—but I still didn't link it to fibroids. I noticed that my girth was increasing, and I mean really increasing. My waist was expanding and my abdomen was protruding. But I attributed that to getting older and gaining weight. I must have been in denial. Also around that point I changed gynecologists. When I got my annual exam that year, he said that he could feel quite a number of fibroids and asked if I was experiencing any pain. I was a little bit startled and told him that I wasn't having any pain. But my doctor was concerned and ordered an ultrasound. The technician who did it [the ultrasound] alarmed me when she said, "You're really growing quite a fruit basket in there." They were huge. I could see them on the screen. Five were growing outside of my uterus and there were multiple fibroids inside as well, too numerous to count. I was shocked. I honestly could not feel them and outside of the urinary frequency and my expanding waistline, I really didn't have any symptoms to complain about.

My gynecologist called in another doctor to consult on my case. And this doctor, who also examined me, said he had never seen fibroids so large and he couldn't believe that I wasn't having more dramatic symptoms. He asked me if I was having this symptom or that symptom and I kept saying, "No, sorry. No. Not that one, either." Then he would say, "Are you sure that you are not in pain?" And I kept saying, "No." There wasn't even a twinge of pain. Now that I think back on it, one of the reasons the fibroids had the opportunity to grow to be so large was because I wasn't feeling any pain. I wasn't experiencing any excessive bleeding, either. I had normal periods. I wasn't having bowel problems. To tell the truth, I felt okay, just fine; maybe a little thicker around the middle, and always racing to the bathroom, but otherwise just fine.

Around this time, partially because of the doctors' reaction and partially because of what I saw on the ultrasound, I started thinking about alternatives to hysterectomy. I knew about uterine artery embolization and thought that would be the best way to go. [Editor's Note: *Uterine artery embolization* is a radiological procedure in which a catheter is introduced through the femoral artery and guided to the uterine arteries, which supply blood to the uterus and, thus, to the fibroids. Tiny micro-particles are then injected into the uterine arteries to block the flow of blood to abnormal growths, which, in turn, causes them to shrink.]

But my doctor told me that I had far too many fibroids for that procedure and that it would not be successful in my case. That didn't stop me from searching for an alternative. I read everything that I could find on fibroids. But again, it was just like it was when the doctors kept asking about symptoms they thought I should have. Books listed lots of symptoms, too. And I kept thinking: "I don't have this one; I don't have that one." I didn't have any that seemed to warrant a hysterectomy. I was trying to hold out because I knew that when I reached menopause they should shrink. But my doctor told me that due to the size to which mine had grown, they probably would remain fairly large after menopause.

And he was right. As time wore on the urinary frequency worsened. I was having an extreme problem with it. The fibroids had begun pressing on my bladder and they were pressing on the spine and my coccyx area. My doctor recommended a hysterectomy and I agreed that it would be best. I was 53 when he performed the surgery. I had to have an abdominal operation because of the large number of fibroids, their bulkiness, and the fact that so many had grown on the outside of the uterus. During the operation, the doctors took pictures of the fibroids. My doctor later showed them to me and, as suspected, they were very large. I was surprised that so many had crowded into such a small space and had grown to be so large. Taking pictures is not unusual; surgeons do it all the time for all kinds of operations and a hysterectomy is no exception. They take pictures for the chart when they remove [structures] from your body. I didn't have any complications from the surgery. I was up walking immediately afterward and healed quickly. But I took six weeks off from work to recuperate. I healed so well, you can hardly tell where I had surgery.

Right after my hysterectomy and for a few months afterward, I'd say about six months after surgery, I was able to drink as much water as I wanted—whenever I wanted—and did not have the problem with urgency. It was such a great feeling to be able to do that, to drink a glass of water and not have to run to the nearest bathroom. But now it's coming back. The urgency is there when I drink water and it's so strong an urge that I have to go right away. I think my muscles may be weakening and it is getting to a point that it's more like incontinence than urinary frequency. I wear liners and monitor very closely the amount of fluids I take in to avoid any kind of embarrassment. [The patient noted during this interview that she had not yet seen her physician about urinary incontinence.]

I know that this is something I will have to cope with. I don't lift patients any more. I know that kind of pressure can force the urge to urinate. In my current position, I monitor patients when they come to the hospital. I review their charts for medical necessity and help determine whether they should be hospitalized or be treated as an outpatient. I also monitor my own condition and know that I will need further treatment for a problem that could not be permanently fixed by a hysterectomy.

—Hysterectomy Patient

PART ONE

Basic Facts About Hysterectomy

Why is a hysterectomy performed?

How effective are less-invasive alternatives?

What are the different ways in which a hysterectomy is performed?

More . . .

1. My doctor has recommended a hysterectomy, but I understand there are pros and cons to the surgery. What should I know about the big picture?

Despite concerns dating back 40 years that far too many women undergo hysterectomies, the procedure remains the most common non-obstetrical form of surgery performed on women in the United States today. Hysterectomy is surpassed only by Caesarean section in the number of operations women undergo annually. Statistics from the Centers for Disease Control and Prevention (CDC) show that an estimated one in four women will have her uterus—and very likely her ovaries—removed by the time she reaches her 60th birthday. While the overall rate at which the surgery is performed has decreased significantly since the 1980s, rates vary further by age, region, and level of education.

Hysterectomy is surpassed only by Caesarean section in the number of operations women undergo annually.

Not only are women slightly younger and more likely to undergo hysterectomies in some parts of the United States than others, statistics show that those with only a high school education are more likely to have a hysterectomy than those who attended college or completed more advanced degrees. The reasoning behind the latter suggests that women who are better educated are more likely to avail themselves of information about alternative procedures and to actively pursue those treatments. Nevertheless, statistics provide broad assessments, painting scenarios in generalities that may have very little in common with your individual circumstances, and as such, may not pertain to you. Hysterectomy is a surgery that has remained an inescapable fact of life for countless women in the United States regardless of social class, race, and level of education.

If you have a condition that has not been controlled by less invasive methods and your physician is recommending a hysterectomy, you will want to know as much as possible about the procedure. On the other hand, if you think the surgery has been recommended as your only choice and you would like to know about a less drastic alternative, then you will want to investigate your options, seek a second opinion, and find the best way to alleviate your medical problem by avoiding a major operation that requires weeks of recuperation.

Basically, the term **hysterectomy** refers to the removal of the uterus, which is also called the womb. Of course, depending on the diagnosis, other reproductive structures might also be removed to effectively treat a specific condition. In addition to the uterus, the procedure can include the cervix, the fallopian tubes, and the ovaries. You may have heard the term **total hysterectomy**, which on first blush seems to refer to the surgical removal of all reproductive tract structures. Instead, it means the uterus and cervix. The surgery that usually is performed for pelvic-area disease other than cancer is a **subtotal hysterectomy**, the removal of the pear-shaped uterus.

Hysterectomy is a form of surgery that has its roots in a centuries-old past; its very name recalls Greek origins: *hystera*, which refers to the womb, and *hysterikos*, the Greek word for hysteria. The term hysterectomy stems from the ancient notion that women were more likely than men to lose control emotionally and become hysterical. Removing the womb, the ancients believed, delivered women from the source of their madness. It took centuries for such ill-founded beliefs to fade.

hysterectomy
The surgical removal of the uterus (the womb).

total hysterectomy
The surgical removal of the uterus and cervix.

subtotal hysterectomy
The surgical removal of the pear-shaped uterus; this surgery usually is performed for pelvic-area disease other than cancer.

3

Today, hysterectomy is one choice for the treatment of major reproductive system disorders, but it exists increasingly in an arena of less invasive medical procedures, many involving groundbreaking technological innovations. Still, when medically warranted, a hysterectomy has helped to dramatically change lives that once were dominated by pain, bleeding, and disability.

Several key intellectual advances over the past 25 years have had an impact on hysterectomies. Newer, less radical alternatives have helped force a 20% decline in the number of hysterectomies that are performed annually in the United States. There has been a keener understanding of the psychological impact that a hysterectomy can have—both good and bad—on women who undergo the surgery. For instance, when the procedure ends abnormal uterine bleeding, eliminates the further threat of cancer, or frees patients from the source of excruciating pain, then its psychological boost is said to be immeasurable. On the other hand, because the surgery ends the ability to reproduce, for those women who held hopes of bearing children, its impact can be psychologically difficult.

2. Why is a hysterectomy performed?

Several medical conditions have long been associated with hysterectomy: **uterine fibroids**, which are benign tumors that can cause severe abnormal bleeding and extreme pain (discussed more fully in Part 4); **endometriosis**, a disorder in which uterine tissue inappropriately implants itself outside of the uterus and throughout the pelvic area, triggering severe pain and irregular menstrual bleeding (see Part 5); **uterine prolapse**, a condition in which the uterus (and in some

uterine fibroids

Benign tumors that can cause severe abnormal bleeding and extreme pain; also known as fibromyoma, leiomyoma, and myoma. May trigger heavy menstrual bleeding, disabling cramps, unpredictable bleeding between periods, and may underlie serious anemia and exhaustion.

endometriosis

A reproductive system disorder where tissue from the inner lining of the uterus grows in places it should not be. Endometrial tissue can implant itself anywhere in the pelvic area (including the ovaries, the bladder, and even the large intestine), leading to scar tissue and pain during sexual intercourse and bowel movements. Some patients report a constant dull pain in the abdomen, and an escalation in the degree of pain during menstruation.

instances the bladder as well) drops from its normal position and protrudes into the vagina (see Part 7); **pelvic inflammatory disease**, which results from overwhelming infections (see Part 8); and **cancer**, which can affect any of the pelvic structures (see Part 9). Certainly there are other conditions for which the surgery is performed, but the primary one in the United States is uterine fibroid tumors, growths that sometimes lead to such profuse bleeding women must be treated in hospital emergency rooms. Cancer generally is perceived to be the strongest reason to perform the operation and also is the condition for which there are few alternative procedures. A more detailed look at the diagnoses necessitating hysterectomy is discussed throughout this book.

3. What are the long-term side effects of a hysterectomy? Are there ways I can avoid them or keep them at bay?

Although some women have reported long-term depression, sexual dysfunction, and fatigue following their surgeries, the most obvious long-term effects of a hysterectomy are an end to fertility, menstruation, and childbearing in women of reproductive age. The goal set by most physicians performing hysterectomies on patients of reproductive age is to leave the ovaries intact when at all possible, thus preserving hormone production.

Despite physicians' hopes of maintaining patients' capacity to produce hormones, there are cases when doing so is impossible. For example, when cancer is present the ovaries must be removed; the same may hold true in certain instances of endometriosis when

uterine prolapse

Also known as pelvic relaxation, this condition occurs when the ligaments that hold the uterus and/or bladder in place loosen. Severe weakening may allow the organ(s) to protrude through the vagina.

pelvic inflammatory disease (PID)

Acute or chronic inflammation of female pelvic structures (endometrium, uterine tubes, pelvic peritoneum) due to infection (gonorrhea, chlamydia, and other organisms). If untreated, PID can result in scarring and infertility.

cancer

Any malignant development caused by abnormal and uncontrolled growth of cells. Some cancers grow rapidly and invade surrounding tissues and organs; others are more indolent and grow slowly.

oophorectomy
Removal of the ovaries; can trigger the immediate onset of menopause and menopausal symptoms, including: hot flashes, night sweats, mood swings, vaginal dryness, and short-term memory loss.

estrogen
A hormone formed by the ovaries, the placenta during pregnancy, and, to a lesser extent, by fat cells with the aid of an enzyme called aromatase. Estrogen stimulates secondary sex characteristics, such as the growth of breasts, and exerts systemic effects (i.e., growth and maturation of long bones, and control of the menstrual cycle).

You definitely will want to know if taking estrogen is right for you.

the ovaries are excessively overcome by endometrial implants and scarring, or in cases of pervasive pelvic inflammatory disease. Removing the ovaries (a surgical procedure known as **oophorectomy**) can trigger the immediate onset of menopause and its potent symptoms: hot flashes, night sweats, mood swings, vaginal dryness, and short-term memory loss, to name a few. Surgically induced menopause is sudden and dramatic. The long-term side effects of removing the ovaries can include an increased risk of osteoporosis (bone loss), heart disease, decreased muscle mass, a gradual change in the distribution of body fat, and a loss of libido (sexual drive).

It is possible to reduce the intensity of some of those side effects by replacing the **estrogen** that you are no longer able to produce on your own. Your doctor can write a prescription for estrogen replacement therapy. Estrogen replacement, however, is not without its own set of risks and may trigger a host of concerns that you will want to discuss with your health care provider. You definitely will want to know if taking estrogen is right for you.

Rigorous clinical trials have shown an increased risk for strokes and abnormal blood clotting, not only among women on estrogen therapy, but also for those taking another type of **hormone replacement therapy** in which pills contain both estrogen and progestin. This type of hormone therapy, commonly called HRT, is the kind prescribed to women who still have a uterus. For them, estrogen-only pills would greatly increase the risk of uterine cancer. These women still are not home free: HRT elevates the risk of breast cancer. Results from the Women's Health Initiative (WHI), a massive study of health concerns involving post-menopausal women, did not find an elevated breast cancer risk in women who had undergone a hysterectomy and who took estrogen-only pills.

The analysis of nearly 11,000 women who were randomly assigned to take either a daily estrogen pill or a placebo found that participants who took the hormone faced no greater danger of breast cancer than those taking dummy pills. However, WHI researchers found in a separate arm of their research that women on estrogen therapy had an elevated risk of deep vein thrombosis, a potentially fatal clotting condition in which a blood clot can travel through the bloodstream and lodge in a lung or cause a stroke. Smokers should be especially aware of the risks associated with abnormal clotting. If you want to take estrogen pills after your ovaries have been removed, then you will have to break your habit. It is important to discuss these matters thoroughly with your physician, especially if there are any issues suggesting that estrogen therapy could prove riskier than usual for you. Also, if you are around the age of 50 and nearing a natural menopause, you may not want to invite the risks inherent in taking estrogen pills, and may choose to avoid hormone therapy altogether. Again, even this choice is something that you will want to discuss with your doctor. Prevailing medical wisdom suggests a cautious approach to estrogen therapy, despite the news that estrogen-only pills do not increase the risk of breast cancer. Women should take the lowest dose to control hot flashes and other symptoms for the shortest time possible.

As ominous as the discussion has seemed so far, none of this is aimed at suggesting that estrogen replacement is a proposition entirely filled with risks. The therapy may have a long-term dividend, at least in one

hormone replacement therapy (HRT)
Medication containing one or more female hormones. Most often HRT is used to treat symptoms of menopause (hot flashes, vaginal dryness, mood swings, sleep disorders, and decreased sexual desire). Estrogen replacement therapy is a form of HRT that includes only the estrogen hormone.

key respect: Estrogen has the capacity to help prevent the development of osteoporosis, a disabling condition in which bones can easily fracture.

Meanwhile, the long-term side effects of hysterectomy are still being studied because they have raised serious research questions. Scientists are asking whether the surgery causes urinary incontinence in some women? Can a hysterectomy increase the likelihood of chronic constipation? Can diminished sexual response be a long-term side effect of the operation? While the answer is yes to all of those questions, none of the problems are pervasive among women who have had a hysterectomy, but they are common enough to have raised concern.

urinary incontinence

An inability to prevent the excretion of urine.

For example, with respect to **urinary incontinence**, there have been mixed results from studies investigating the surgery's impact on bladder function. Some studies have found a link between the surgery and urinary incontinence, while others have not. Among those studies that have pinpointed a link, doctors say damage occurred to pelvic nerves during the operation or to pelvic support structures. Either way, bladder function was adversely affected. Surgical injury is not restricted to the most invasive form of hysterectomy. Urinary tract injuries have been known to occur with a minimally invasive hysterectomy in which the uterus is removed through the vagina. Researchers have been working on nerve-sparing surgical techniques as well as ways to avoid urinary tract injury. (A more complete discussion on hysterectomy and urinary incontinence is in Question #99.)

Although not very common, another possible long-term side effect is slow-propulsion constipation, a disorder that also is known as slow-transit constipation.

The American Society of Colon and Rectal Surgeons lists hysterectomy as one of many possible causes of this chronic condition and attributes the problem to localized damage to pelvic nerves sustained during surgery. Yet even with an established link between this chronic form of constipation and hysterectomy, doctors point to numerous other causes, which can include the use or abuse of certain medications, particularly opioid drugs; anticonvulsants, and calcium- or aluminum-containing antacids, among other medications. Such constipation also can occur as a consequence of diabetes and in certain anxiety disorders. Slow-propulsion constipation is treatable in many cases through simple dietary changes. Finally, some women have reported diminished sexual response as a post-hysterectomy side effect, something they say also diminished their quality of life. (Sexual issues are discussed in greater detail in Question #14.)

4. How effective are less-invasive alternatives?

There are therapeutic options for many reproductive system disorders that once were treated exclusively by hysterectomy. Today, women have more options than they did just a decade ago. Conservative techniques and procedures can effectively treat reproductive-organ problems without resorting to hysterectomy. With the exception of cancer, physicians begin by recommending alternative treatments to patients. If you are told that you need a hysterectomy for a non-cancerous condition but are not first told of alternative therapies, then it may be wise to seek a second opinion. The American College of Obstetrics and Gynecology, the leading professional organization of OB/GYN physicians, states in both its patient- and physician-education materials

Today, women have more options than they did just a decade ago.

that, "hysterectomy should be performed only for medical reasons, and only after alternative options have been discussed and explored with the patient."

Alternative treatments can be as simple as common pain relief medications, such as ibuprofen, naproxen, and even enteric-coated aspirin. Other medications, such as birth control pills, are also very familiar. Additional treatments, such as various forms of hormone-based medications, can be used for certain disorders to induce a pseudo-menopausal state. These drugs are administered over several months, which allows time for symptoms of your underlying condition to subside. In the best-case scenario, these medications can force the disorder into retreat. Overall, the list of alternative treatments has grown substantially over the years and now includes many high-tech procedures. Lasers can be used against some conditions. Blood vessels that supply bothersome fibroids can be blocked with the infusion of tiny "microspheres." By obstructing blood flow into the fibroids, the growths are forced to shrink. Fertility-sparing surgeries for several other types of reproductive system disorders (including fibroids) can provide relief from abnormal bleeding or pain while helping you avoid a hysterectomy.

Certainly, the aim here is not to give the impression that conservative procedures are completely free of risks and disappointments. Alternatives to hysterectomy come with their own set of drawbacks. Fertility-sparing surgeries may not be successful and attempts to end excessive bleeding through drug therapy may not work. You as a patient may even become frustrated by the treatments when the results do not seem immediate. Still, when turning to alternative procedures, the goal is to

maintain fertility and to put off—forever if possible—
the need for a dramatically more invasive solution.
While on the subject of alternative procedures, you may
find it noteworthy that the results of numerous studies
have shown that alternative treatments tend to be less
expensive, less debilitating, and less likely to cause a loss
of productivity due to weeks spent recuperating. Recuperation after alternative procedures are significantly
shorter compared with the month to six weeks spent in
recuperation after a hysterectomy.

5. Given the growing number of alternate procedures, could hysterectomy become passé?

Even in light of a 20% decline in the number of hysterectomies performed over the past quarter-century,
which has been attributed to the increasing number of
successful alternative treatments for female reproductive disorders, an estimated 650,000 to 675,000
women still undergo the operation annually in the
United States, according to data from the Centers for
Disease Control (CDC). Indeed, more hysterectomies
are performed in the United States than in any other
Western nation. A study by the Agency for Healthcare
Research and Quality (AHRQ) found that, 5 in every
1,000 women in the United States undergo the operation each year compared with fewer than 3 in every
1,000 in Great Britain and fewer than 2 in every 1,000
in Norway. On the whole, European nations report
substantially lower hysterectomy rates than the United
States, a country where an estimated $5 billion in
health care costs are spent on the surgery annually.

6. Are American physicians more likely to "believe" in hysterectomies?

Hysterectomy is neither a belief system nor a philosophy. It is a surgical procedure requiring a great deal of skill, performed by physicians who are specifically trained to treat conditions of the female reproductive system. But that does not mean all doctors are comfortable with the relatively high number of women who have the operation yearly in the United States. In a report produced by the U.S. Food and Drug Administration that examined alternatives to hysterectomy, Dr. Anthony Scialli (Georgetown University Medical Center, Washington, D.C.) said there are strong reasons to support the surgery in certain instances. "There are cases where hysterectomy is the only option," Scialli is quoted in the report. "But I think we perform too many hysterectomies. It's a matter of American gynecologists being accustomed to performing a hysterectomy and American women being accustomed to getting one based on their mother or other female relative having one. The one thing in favor of a hysterectomy is that it works for abnormal bleeding—but it should be the last step not the first step."

7. What are the different ways in which a hysterectomy is performed?

The surgery can be performed either through an abdominal incision or vaginally. Those are your choices. If you are to have the surgery, then you'll want to thoroughly discuss with your physician why a specific surgical method is being recommended. Your surgeon will examine you, evaluate your level of disease, and then recommend the method that will be most effective in the treatment of your condition. **Abdominal surgeries** generally are chosen for fibroids of relatively large size, certain cases involving endometriosis, and for any form of cancer (ovarian, endometrial, or cervical). Numerous studies have shown that for non-cancerous conditions, doctors should strive for **vaginal surgeries** (removing the uterus through the vagina; see Question #8) when at all possible. There is more than one technique that can be employed to accomplish this task, which will be explained below.

First, it is important to underscore that the way in which your operation is performed can have a bearing on the amount of time you spend recuperating. Abdominal surgeries (which are performed through an incision similar to that for a Caesarean section) are associated with longer recovery periods, more manipulation of other abdominal structures during surgery (your intestines get jostled a bit), and there is a greater degree of post-operative pain. Recovery can take up to six weeks. The majority of hysterectomies performed in the United States are abdominal procedures.

On the plus side, the abdominal operation allows your surgeon a keen view of the uterus and other reproductive organs and sufficient space to remove large fibroids, which sometimes can reach the size of a grapefruit or be even larger. An abdominal hysterectomy, nevertheless, will leave a scar. With vaginal procedures, weeks are eliminated from the recovery period—the recovery takes about a month—and your bowel function returns sooner because there is far less interference with your intestines during surgery. Generally, the overall surgery is less painful. That said, the National Uterine Fibroid Foundation, a nonprofit information clearinghouse based in Colorado, estimates that up to 144 million work hours

abdominal surgeries

Type of surgical procedure performed through an incision similar to the kind made for a Caesarean section.

vaginal surgeries

Type of surgery that removes the uterus through the vagina.

The majority of hysterectomies performed in the United States are abdominal procedures.

are lost annually to recuperation from hysterectomies, regardless of how they are performed. Through its Web site, the Foundation promotes awareness about the number of hysterectomies performed in the United States, especially for uterine fibroids, and underscores that women need to know about less invasive alternatives.

8. My physician is recommending a vaginal hysterectomy. What should I know about this procedure?

Vaginal hysterectomies are less debilitating than abdominal procedures. They can be performed in one of two ways: conventionally or with the aid of a laparoscope. In the conventional procedure, your surgeon makes a cut (called an incision) at the top of the vagina. Through this opening, the surgeon can cut and tie off ligaments and blood vessels. During this process, the fallopian tubes are also disconnected from the uterus, but left in place. The uterus is then freed and removed through the vagina.

laparoscope

A very small, thin surgical instrument that allows inspection of the abdominal organs through a tiny camera attached to the device.

A more advanced surgical technique involves the use of a **laparoscope**, an instrument that allows your physician to inspect abdominal organs through a tiny camera that is part of the device. The laparoscope is inserted through a small incision near the navel. This type of an operation often is informally referred to as *keyhole surgery*, owing to the tiny incision through which instruments are inserted. The procedure also requires vaginal surgery and hence is known as a laparoscopically assisted vaginal hysterectomy. When a laparoscope is used, the hysterectomy is then known as laparoscopic-assisted vaginal hysterectomy (LAVH).

About 10% of hysterectomies performed in the United States are laparoscopic-assisted. This form of surgery is considered to be far less traumatic and the amount of time devoted to recovery is lessened as a result.

A study by the Agency for Healthcare Research and Quality (AHRQ) showed that in the 1990s the number of laparoscopic-assisted hysterectomies increased 30-fold, a trend that is strongly influencing how some surgeons are performing the operation now. However, the AHRQ also underscored that abdominal hysterectomy remains the most common procedure in the United States, accounting for 63% of all hysterectomies. In France and Australia, by comparison, up to 50% of hysterectomy patients undergo operations that are performed vaginally.

9. What is the average age for hysterectomy? Does region play a role in hysterectomy?

Naturally, age varies among women undergoing hysterectomies each year in the United States, but government data show that approximately 55% of those who have the procedure are between the ages of 35 and 49. Within that group, women between the ages of 40 and 45 comprise the largest number of those who have the operation. Age has a strong relationship to hysterectomy because of the types of medical conditions that are most likely to occur during specific points in a woman's reproductive life.

For example, smaller proportions of women who undergo the procedure are older than 55 or younger than 30. Women in their mid-50s and older are more likely than younger women to have the surgery for some form of reproductive-tract cancer, which may include ovarian, cervical, or uterine cancer.

Geographic region is an additional factor underlying the surgery's prevalence. For example, CDC statistics indicate that women who live in the South not only are more likely to undergo a hysterectomy than women who live in other parts of the country, they usually are younger than women elsewhere when they have the procedure. Hysterectomy rates are lowest on the West Coast and in the Northeast, particularly in New York, which has the lowest rate of all 50 states and the District of Columbia. The average age of Southern women at the time of surgery is 41.6 compared with 47.7 for women in other parts of the country. Of course, there are no hard and fast rules regarding age and region. A woman living in California is as likely to undergo a hysterectomy at age 35 as is one living in Georgia, depending on each individual's diagnosis, symptoms, degree of discomfort, and personal choice. However, of the top ten states reporting the highest rates of the operation, seven are located in the Southeast.

10. When should I consider a hysterectomy?

A hysterectomy, generally, is not an operation that must be performed immediately unless the diagnosis is cancer, uterine hemorrhage, intractable pain, or an obstetrical emergency. Therefore, you have time to thoroughly discuss the operation with your physicians and even to ask whether there may still be a chance that an alternative to hysterectomy might better address your reproductive system disorder. If the answer to that question is no, and when symptoms have continued unabated despite earlier treatment through an alternative to hysterectomy (and the consensus opinion of your physicians is a recommendation of hysterectomy), then the surgery may be your best option. Again, the primary reasons for the surgery are: cancer; obstetrical emergencies; uterine prolapse; excessive bleeding that leads to severe anemia and exhaustion; or intractable pain.

If you are not undergoing the surgery for a malignant condition, you may want to ask yourself some tough questions: What would the loss of a uterus, or possibly even both ovaries, mean to you? Do you want to take estrogen replacement therapy (see Question #3)? Are you prepared to handle the psychological fallout from the operation, such as the thought of never being able to bear children if you are of reproductive age?

Of course, you may want to frame your questions in other ways: What new interests can I pursue once I am freed from excessive bleeding and pain? How much happier will I be when I am no longer worried about unpredictable bleeding? Another thought to keep in mind if you are strongly considering the surgery is your time spent recuperating from it. Hysterectomy is considered major surgery and at least a month or more is needed for recovery. Can you be away from work for six weeks, which is the standard amount of time for recovery from an abdominal operation? Finally, you may want to be honest with yourself and ask whether you have tried every possible conservative approach before consenting to invasive surgery.

11. Is a hysterectomy covered by insurance?

Many insurers classify the surgery as elective unless it is being performed for cancer, an obstetrical emergency, or uterine hemorrhage. Some insurers also balk at covering a hysterectomy without the benefit of a second opinion. If this happens to you, it means that another physician will probably have to evaluate your case and arrive at the same conclusion before your health plan agrees to cover the surgery's expense. Additionally, for anyone who has recently signed on to a new health insurance plan, there may be a rule requiring a waiting period of at least six months before the operation is covered. Waiting may seem unfair, especially if you are experiencing symptoms that you and your physicians believe are best remedied by surgery. Some insurance companies, however, have taken a stance that too many of the operations are performed unnecessarily and that women should seek other, less expensive forms of care. These treatments may include taking pain relief medications or any one of several alternate procedures that do not involve surgery and hospitalization.

Of course, there is a counterpoint to this view: Insurance companies are committed to the bottom line. If there are strong medical reasons that surgery would prove to be in your best interest, you should advocate strongly on your own behalf to receive it.

12. What should I do to prepare for a hysterectomy?

Certainly, you will have had a thorough pelvic examination during which your gynecologist manually inspects the uterus and other reproductive structures. You should also have had imaging tests, such as an **ultrasound** exam, to confirm your diagnosis. For your own peace of mind, you should make certain that you have been well informed about the procedure by your gynecologist and that surgery is warranted in your case. You also should avail yourself of any self-help information to ensure that you understand in lay terms exactly what is to occur surgically, that you know which structure or structures are being removed and, if you are of reproductive age, that you understand you no longer will be fertile or able to menstruate.

If your insurance company requires a second opinion, then you will have the recommendation for a hysterectomy from more than one source. In addition, you probably will also want to make certain that you understand the actual procedure that has been recommended, the method in which the surgery will be performed, and how long you can expect to be recuperating from the surgery. Once those preliminaries are behind you, your doctor will order a series of laboratory tests, which will likely include screens of blood and urine. All hysterectomies are performed in a hospital. They are not in-office procedures. Prior to your operation, you will meet with an anesthesiologist who will explain the type of medications that will be used. You will sign an **informed consent form** for the operation. This is a legal document that explains the purpose of the surgery, and that you have been told about the surgery's details as well as its potential risks and complications.

ultrasound
A type of imaging machine that uses high frequency soundwaves for medical diagnoses.

informed consent form
A legal document that explains any invasive medical procedure, which must be read and signed by the patient in advance. Most forms describe the procedure and indicate that you have been informed of its risks and benefits.

13. Can a hysterectomy affect my sex life?

Some women report varying degrees of sexual dysfunction after a hysterectomy while others report experiencing no side effects whatsoever. Instead, they say that their sex lives improved after hysterectomy because they were no longer inhibited by abnormal uterine bleeding or the excruciating discomfort caused by a large encumbering fibroid, endometriosis, or other pain-producing pelvic condition. Severe pain brought on by reproductive system disorders can severely limit the quality of sexual relationships, and thus make intercourse difficult. When the source of the pain is alleviated, sex then can become more enjoyable.

Sexual function itself is multifaceted. It involves physiological, psychological and complex emotional responses that involve feelings toward your partner, the surroundings in which the sexual encounter occurs, and various notions about the sexual act. Even the level of stress in your life comes into play. Stress can diminish sexual desire. Medical investigations have revealed posthysterectomy difficulties ranging from loss of libido to problems with arousal to loss of orgasmic quality. Some of these factors have very little to do with whether you have a uterus, which is not to diminish the role of the uterus in female sexuality.

The uterus is believed to be involved in a woman's sexual response and contracts during orgasms. For some women, the absence of uterine contractions after a hysterectomy may affect her capacity to enjoy sex. This sense of loss can be a source of great anxiety. But keep in mind sexual response not only is highly variable from one person to another, it is, as noted earlier, very complex. Uterine contractions may not dominate the quality of intercourse for some women. For women who had a type of uterine fibroid known as a **submucosal fibroid**, the loss of uterine contractions may have occurred long before the hysterectomy because the growth tends to distort uterine shape and lessen the organ's ability to contract.

Virtually any kind of pelvic surgery, including hysterectomy, has the potential to affect the nerves and blood vessels that supply the reproductive system. If a hysterectomy is being strongly recommended and you have concerns about sexual dysfunction, it is very important to have a very open discussion with your physician before your surgery to understand how this can be avoided. Sometimes just knowing that your physician is confident and cares about issues that are important to you can help bolster your spirits as you face major surgery. Also, if you have already had the operation and believe you may be experiencing sexual dysfunction related to your surgery, you should discuss the matter with a gynecologist. It cannot be stressed enough that just because the potential exists for nerve and blood vessels to be adversely affected, this does not mean that you will be harmed in any way. That is why talking with your gynecologist is so important.

Just gathering a sense of what the surgery entails beforehand and knowing which structures will be removed can provide you with a stronger idea of what will happen long before you are wheeled into the surgical suite. Medical researchers have only begun to study the full range of complaints women have made about sexual dysfunction following a hysterectomy. They also have begun to better gauge which complaints are most frequently reported. Sometimes the issue may be depression, which can have an effect on

submucous or submucosal fibroid

A type of fibroid tumor that develops directly beneath the surface of the endometrium. The large number of blood vessels on its surface can bleed and trigger pain. These fibroids tend to prevent the uterine muscle's ability to properly contract because they distort the shape and function of the organ; they can grow to a size that obstructs the fallopian tubes and also may distort the uterine lining as they grow, causing menstrual irregularities. They may even become pedunculated and project into the cervix or even the vagina.

your sexual response. If such is the case, then counseling and/or medication may address the problem.

Here is something else that you may want to keep in the forefront of your thoughts: When balanced against reports from women who say their sex lives improved after a hysterectomy, it is clear that sexual dysfunction is not a universal complaint among the vast number of women who have had the surgery. Among those who say their sex lives improved, many point to being free of abnormal bleeding and/or pain, which allowed spontaneity to again become part of their sex lives.

Nevertheless, there are additional concerns involving sexual matters that you will want to make note of if you are having the surgery. Whether your operation is vaginal or abdominal, you will be advised against sexual intercourse for a few weeks after the procedure. Of course, this recommendation for temporary abstinence is for several reasons. Your doctor's chief concern is lowering your risk for infection. In addition, your health care provider wants to ensure that you give your pelvic area enough time to heal properly following the trauma of surgery and the loss of structures that once filled the space. While some women have remarked that they had resumed sexual activity with vigor and enthusiasm after the few weeks of abstinence following their operations, others report discomfort with intercourse. In some patients, the operation can result in scar tissue or even a slight shortening of the vaginal passageway.

If your ovaries are removed, your hormone levels are no longer what they used to be, so your libido may diminish and you may have additional problems with lubrication and vaginal dryness. These issues are not insurmountable, however. Hormones can be prescribed to counteract issues with libido. The medications also can help enhance lubrication and combat vaginal dryness.

As for a shortened vagina, it can be stretched with repeated attempts at intercourse. The vagina is extraordinarily elastic, a fact that you are probably already well aware of if you have ever had a baby. The take-home message here is simple: you can regain a satisfying sex life after a hysterectomy. For some women, the transition from their pre-operative sex lives to the ones after the operation is seamless. In fact, they remark that with the alleviation of problems with chronic bleeding and pain, sex was a welcome alternative. For others, achieving a healthy sex life after hysterectomy may require some effort. But if you and your partner are willing to work through the problem period, it is likely that you will be able to have a healthy sex life after your surgery.

Hormones can be prescribed to counteract issues with libido.

14. Hysterectomy seems to be as much a political issue as it is a medical one. Why are women's health groups so concerned about the surgery?

Hysterectomy has generated intense concern among women's health advocacy groups for nearly a half century and usually for the very obvious reason that it is a major health intervention that hundreds of thousands of women face each year. Concerns about hysterectomy and its necessity are no longer just the turf of women's health groups but also have become a focus of health insurers, physicians, and major medical organizations. Virtually all of them recommend that women first try alternate procedures before agreeing to a hysterectomy when at all possible.

Women's health advocacy groups have long had a very specific aim: to help women make informed decisions about the operation, and to spread the word about alternatives to the surgery. It would be both a disservice and a mistake to define members of these groups as hotheaded militants with political axes to grind. The groups are varied and cut across a wide spectrum of focus and influence. Yes, many women's health advocacy groups have been strongly motivated by the sheer number of hysterectomies performed annually in the United States. Yes, they have openly stated that many, if not most, of the operations might be avoidable, and their concern stems from the vast number of hysterectomies that are performed as elective procedures. Indeed, many believe that if women were better informed about alternatives, perhaps there would be fewer hysterectomies. But bear in mind that it was activism that first helped awaken the public—and the medical community—to the surgery's extreme overuse a generation ago. From these groups' grassroots efforts today, other issues, such as calling attention to the types of subtle post-hysterectomy side effects that may take years or even decades to manifest, have become yet another rallying point.

Years ago, women took aim against what they felt was an insensitive medical community, which they believed viewed the female reproductive system as a useless group of organs once women had finished childbearing or had reached a certain age. Sherrill Sellman, author of the book *Hormone Heresy*, wrote in an essay entitled *Hysterectomy Heresy* that women faced a formidable medical community in the early 1970s. Many doctors felt hysterectomy should be the norm. "The overwhelming conclusion regarding whether every woman who is finished with childbearing should have a hysterectomy was summed up by gynecologist Ralph W. White," Sellman reported in a retrospective of the 1971 meeting of the American College of Obstetrics and Gynecology. "He expressed the members' prevailing attitude of respect for the female womb by proclaiming, 'It's a useless, bleeding, symptom-producing, potential cancer-bearing organ.'"

In the twenty-first century, the Internet has helped women's health organizations evolve beyond the bitter issues of the 1960s and 70s. Women are being invited into online support and discussion groups in which any issue is open to debate. Post-hysterectomy sexual response, incontinence, depression, fatigue, relationship issues, and weight gain—you name it—are all being discussed online. Chat formats on numerous Web sites have allowed women facing hysterectomy to discuss their fears with those who have already undergone the surgery.

Of course, you may ask what these organizations are like. Some groups have broad memberships that are open to women with any type of condition that can lead to a hysterectomy. Other groups are more narrowly focused and deal with a single medical condition that can result in the surgery. For instance, the group may focus its interests on endometriosis, uterine fibroids, or gynecological cancers. While such organizations have an interest in hysterectomy, they also are focused on conveying information about the medical conditions to which they are devoted.

Finally, a group may be quite general in its aim, with its membership composed of women who underwent or who are considering the surgery for any number of reasons. These groups are not concerned about controversies surrounding the surgery, but the way in which women are coping pre- and post-hysterectomy. A prime example of the latter is a group that calls itself *HysterSisters.com*, a Denton, Texas online organization that offers support groups via its Web site. This allows women to discuss their fears and concerns regarding hysterectomy and other, less invasive alternatives. In its published mission statement the group defines itself as "neither anti-hysterectomy nor pro-hysterectomy," which is proof that women's health groups can be concerned about the surgery without taking a political stance. The group does not avoid controversial subjects. Topics such as sexual dysfunction and troubles women have experienced with estrogen replacement therapy after the operation are open to discussion by Web site visitors.

Certainly, this is not to say that women's groups have mellowed and have lost the fire that first helped them draw attention to the surgery and its aftereffects. Groups such as the HERS Foundation (Hysterectomy Educational Resources and Services) based in suburban Philadelphia, take a far stronger position against the surgery and urge women through its Web site and national conferences to avoid hysterectomies when at all possible. The foundation collects data on post-hysterectomy side effects through polling that it conducts. The data are maintained on the foundation's Web site.

For nearly a decade, the foundation sought information on the most common side effects from the surgery by polling women about their experiences. The group noted "personality change" as the number one long-term side effect reported by most women who had undergone a hysterectomy and who responded to the foundation's questionnaire. HERS defines its mission as providing information about "alternatives to, and consequences of, hysterectomy," and urges women to actively seek alternatives to the surgery. The HERS foundation also has called on women to protest unwarranted hysterectomies.

Their battle cry, which would have been considered radical a generation ago, increasingly has found reinforcement in mainstream medicine, which independently has demonstrated through rigorous scientific research that many claims from advocates have been right on target. In a study published in the journal *Obstetrics and Gynecology*, Dr. Michael Broder (a medical researcher at the University of Southern California) reported that 70% of the surgeries were probably recommended inappropriately, and that women who were told they needed to have a hysterectomy could have fared better without the operation. Dr. Broder's study of 500 women who had undergone hysterectomies for non-emergencies also indicated that many of the patients had been inadequately evaluated for the surgery.

In that same vein, the National Uterine Fibroids Foundation (NUFF) has sounded an alarm about a range of problems associated with hysterectomies, from the number of procedures performed annually to the surgery's high-flying costs. The foundation devotes its energies to raising awareness about the high rate of hysterectomies performed for uterine fibroids and maintains a database of statistics about the surgery. It collects information from a variety of sources, such as the Centers for Disease Control and Prevention and the American College of Obstetrics and Gynecology.

The foundation notes that for every 10,000 hysterectomies performed each year in the United States, 11 women die. A total of about 660 deaths a year are attributable to hysterectomy complications, according to the foundation. Among the more than 600,000 hysterectomies performed annually, 60% of patients have their ovaries removed, and more than $5 billion is spent on hormone replacement therapy alone. An additional $5 billion is spent for the surgery itself. Alarms from the NUFF and similar groups have not gone unheard. Some doctors inform their patients about the groups as a source of education.

Advocacy groups and mainstream medicine have found common ground in another area of concern: the need for a greater emphasis on research into new and better methods of treating female reproductive system disorders. Dr. Donna Shoupe (Women's and Children's Hospital in Los Angeles) was among the first physicians to question the wisdom of routinely removing the ovaries of women aged 45 and older during hysterectomies, a practice that was very common as recently as the 1990s (and has yet to fully disappear).

Bilateral oophorectomies (surgical removal of both ovaries) were being performed along with the removal of the uterus based on the belief that women were more likely to develop ovarian cancer as they aged. Removing the ovaries, doctors thought, would reduce the cancer risk. But studies increasingly demonstrate that the ovaries still produce hormones in older women. The new discoveries are flying in the face of conventional wisdom, which generally considered the two glands as having virtually no function after menopause. Some studies now suggest the ovaries play a role well into the later years of life, producing hormones such as testosterone and minute amounts of estrogen for up to 10 years past menopause.

If you do not have cancer or a condition that has severely compromised ovarian function and the recommendation is to remove your ovaries as part of your hysterectomy, you may want to have a long discussion with your physician about the necessity of an oophorectomy.

Many in the women's health advocacy community had long opposed the routine removal of the ovaries in women undergoing hysterectomies. Oophorectomies create an instant need for hormone replacement therapy, a treatment that has proven to be problematic in some women. Often, health care providers must work with them to find the formulation that is most helpful. In addition, routine oophorectomies also overlooked the role that the ovaries play in post-menopausal women.

Studies increasingly demonstrate that the ovaries still produce hormones in older women.

15. Are there any positive factors related to hysterectomy?

Hysterectomy has many positives. In countless instances, hysterectomies have rescued women from life-threatening conditions. For those who have been treated for cancer, there is the relief knowing that the cancer has been removed and a major step has been taken toward restoring health. There also is a feeling of relief among women whose lives were dominated by excessive blood loss, which led to anemia and its accompanying fatigue. And, there is a sense of relief from the intractable pain produced by endometriosis, large fibroids, or any other reproductive organ abnormality. Some women have even said their surgeries afforded them newfound freedom because their lives were no longer limited by a chronic medical condition. To reiterate, though, hysterectomy generally is necessary only for disorders that are life-threatening, such as cancer, an obstetrical emergency, excessive bleeding, or severe uterine prolapse. For any other reason, the surgery is elective.

PART TWO

Psychological and Emotional Impact of Abnormal Uterine Bleeding and Pain: Is Hysterectomy Always the Right Solution?

I have persistent bleeding and fatigue.
Are my problems age-related? Will a hysterectomy
solve my problem?

I have heard that a hysterectomy can cause long-term
depression. Is this true?

Can my gynecologist treat depression?

More . . .

16. I have persistent bleeding and fatigue. Are my problems age-related? Will a hysterectomy solve my problem?

Abnormal uterine bleeding is a formidable problem among women of reproductive age and is the reason for millions of visits to gynecologists annually in the United States. An estimated 1 in every 5 visits to U.S. gynecologists is for **abnormal uterine bleeding**, a disorder that can be caused by any one of several underlying reproductive system conditions. According to a report in the journal *American Family Physician*, about 20.1 million visits are made to gynecologists annually and an estimated 25% of gynecologic surgeries (hysterectomies and fertility-sparing procedures) are performed to address problems of abnormal uterine bleeding. A seriously low red-blood cell count, called **anemia**, affects two thirds of women with abnormal uterine bleeding. If you have become seriously depressed because of your condition, the psychological impact may seem amplified and burdensome because of the fatigue and exhaustion that can occur as a result of a low red-blood cell count.

Abnormal bleeding can be frequent, sustained, or totally unpredictable. It can be an issue that has minimal impact on your overall health and is cleared up quickly, or it may become an episodic but nagging medical problem that can last for years. For some women, abnormal bleeding occurs as spotting between menstrual periods. For others it is heavy bleeding during their periods (**menstruation**), requiring very frequent changes of tampons or protective pads. For still others, particularly those at the end of their reproductive years, excessive uterine bleeding can seem as if menstrual periods never end, the blood loss serving as the underlying cause of anemia, fatigue, and a dimin-

abnormal uterine bleeding

A disorder caused by any one of several underlying reproductive system conditions; characterized by excessive bleeding and/or blood clots that may lead to anemia.

anemia

A disorder in which there is a low red blood cell count; red blood cells carry less oxygen. Anemia can result in fatigue and exhaustion. If untreated may prove life-threatening.

menstruation

A discharge of blood, secretions, and tissue fragments from the uterus at regular intervals, usually after ovulation.

ished quality of life. If you are thoroughly saturating a tampon or pad every hour throughout your periods, then your bleeding is probably excessive.

When bleeding is excessive, it can put limits on life's spontaneity and freedom. It also can have an adverse effect on relationships with friends and family members, your sex life, and the ability to function effectively in the workplace. Frequent absenteeism because of abnormal uterine bleeding can be a cause of losing one's employment, and job loss even without an underlying medical condition is a major reason for depression. In instances when heavy bleeding is persistent, it can lead to fainting. But it cannot be emphasized more strongly that, even if your abnormal bleeding is chronic, a hysterectomy is not inevitable, no matter where you are in your reproductive life. For very young women, the prospects of hysterectomy do not enter the discussion unless circumstances are life-threatening. A thorough medical examination will be performed to find out the specific cause or causes of the bleeding.

Your doctor has a number of conservative treatments to offer that can effectively treat excessive bleeding. It is only when bleeding is unresponsive to conservative treatment, or in instances when severe bleeding is life-threatening that hysterectomy enters discussions between you and your physician. Your doctor's first move will be to run a series of tests to reach a diagnosis. You may undergo a diagnostic procedure called **hysteroscopy**, which involves the use of a telescopic instrument to inspect the uterus. There are several solutions which may be used to distend the uterus. The procedure may be performed in the office under local anesthesia, or in the hospital under general anesthesia. The uterus is

hysteroscopy
A diagnostic procedure that uses a telescopic instrument to inspect the uterus.

visible on a screen during this procedure, so you are able to see inside your uterus as your gynecologist conducts an inspection. A small tissue sample is taken during the procedure, which is sent to a laboratory for examination.

Some doctors may use a diagnostic procedure called **dilation and curettage (D&C)**. This diagnostic procedure can be performed under general anesthesia or an **epidural**, which means that nerves will be numbed from the waist down. Your doctor will dilate the cervix and then, with a spoon-shaped instrument called a curette, scrape the uterus and send a tissue specimen to a laboratory for examination. For some women, a D&C proves therapeutic and ends abnormal bleeding. Few doctors rely on a D&C as a therapeutic measure because bleeding problems can return.

You may also find it helpful to have a stronger grasp on why abnormal bleeding occurs. Sometimes diagnosed as a condition called **dysfunctional uterine bleeding (DUB)**, your health care provider will probably suspect it when you are not pregnant (because pregnancy can trigger bleeding) or you have not been taking hormone-based medications (which can cause spotting). About 70% to 90% of DUB cases are typified by menstrual periods that are **anovulatory**, which means that an egg was not produced. Releasing an egg is an important step in the menstrual cycle because each step in the cycle leads to the next. It is synchronous, based on interdependence and timing. Any miscue affects all of the steps that follow. As women age, the ovaries begin shutting down egg production, and an increasing number of the periods are anovulatory. The lack of egg production affects the overall character of menstrual cycles and can lead to abnormal bleeding.

dilation and curettage (D&C)

A diagnostic procedure performed when the woman is under general anesthesia or an epidural; the cervix is dilated, and then with a spoon-shaped instrument called a curette, the uterus is scraped. The resulting tissue specimen is sent to a laboratory for analysis.

epidural

A procedure in which nerves are numbed from the waist down.

dysfunctional uterine bleeding (DUB)

Excessive uterine bleeding.

anovulatory

Menstrual periods in which an egg is not produced.

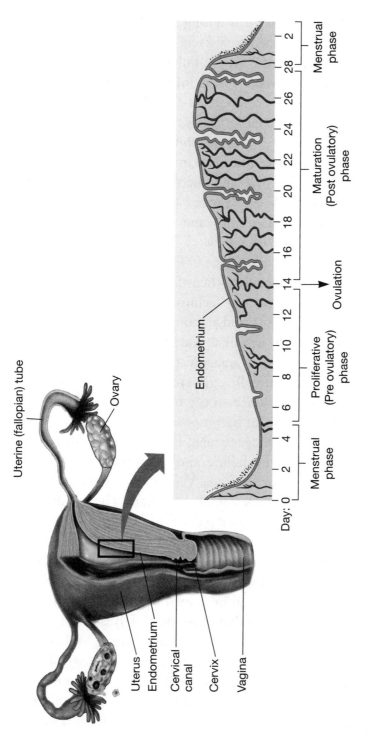

The menstrual cycle

35

When all is normal during the first 14 days, the first half of your menstrual cycle is dominated by estrogen, which causes the uterine lining to thicken. During this phase, egg production is inhibited by estrogen as the hormone goes about its job of building up the endometrium and prepares for pregnancy. When ovulation occurs with the ripening of an egg, the hormone called **progesterone** kicks in to stop uterine thickening by changing the endometrial lining to prepare for pregnancy. When a pregnancy doesn't happen, progesterone secretion stops and the uterine lining breaks down as menstrual flow.

In **perimenopause**, when the ovaries no longer function as efficient egg factories, some women find that their cycle can't budge from its first phase. Bleeding can become irregular and profuse because progesterone, estrogen's antagonist, never arrives to perform its duties. Normally, eggs are produced in the ovary by **follicle cells**. Once an egg bursts from the follicle, the follicle's remnant becomes known as the *corpus luteum* and secretes progesterone. However, when there is no egg, there is no follicle and when there is no follicle, there is no *corpus luteum*. Without a *corpus luteum* there can be no progesterone secretion. The result is an absence of the second half of the menstrual cycle.

Dysfunctional uterine bleeding has important relationships to age for more reasons than one. About half of all cases of DUB occur in women who are in their mid-40s or who are somewhat older. But DUB isn't just a problem of aging ovaries. In young women, a hormonal imbalance typified by low levels of progesterone can lead to bouts of irregular bleeding that are indistinguishable from those experienced by perimenopausal women. Among adolescents and even women in their

progesterone

A sex hormone that prepares the uterus for pregnancy.

perimenopause

A stage in a woman's life when the ovaries no longer function as in youth; precursor of menopause.

follicle cells

A type of cell located in the ovary that produces eggs.

20s, menstrual periods may not have become regulated; in older women the irregular bleeding is due to increasing degrees of ovarian failure.

Your health care provider will want to conduct a thorough medical examination because symptoms of DUB are very similar to other causes of abnormal bleeding. In fact, DUB can occur simultaneously with other causes of bleeding. Your gynecologist will ask you a number of questions as she or he documents your medical history, taking note of how your menstrual cycles functioned from puberty to the present. Having an understanding of your cycle's history will help your doctor to analyze the character of your current menstrual cycles. Does your period last longer than seven days? Is the bleeding soaking a pad or tampon every hour? Do you have bleeding between periods? Are your periods appearing more frequently than an ordinary menstrual cycle? Heavy menstrual bleeding within a normal cycle is called **menorrhagia**, and this can prove to be a symptom of DUB. Menorrhagia also can be a symptom of other disorders, which will be discussed in greater detail below. In addition to menorrhagia, there are other terms to define an abnormal menstrual cycle. **Metrorrhagia** refers to bleeding between menstrual periods. **Polymenorrhea** refers to periods that occur far too frequently, usually within a cycle of less than 21 days.

Among women in their 40s and early 50s, bleeding may be related to any one of several causes beyond the lack of ovulation that results in dysfunctional uterine bleeding. Uterine fibroids are a major reason for excessive bleeding. As women near the end of their reproductive years, fibroids begin to soften and bleed, sometimes very profusely, producing what may seem like an endless men-

menorrhagia

Heavy menstrual bleeding within a normal cycle; may be a symptom of dysfunctional uterine bleeding.

metrorrhagia

Bleeding between menstrual periods; may be a symptom of dysfunctional uterine bleeding.

polymenorrhea

Menstrual periods that occur far too frequently, usually within a cycle of less than 21days; may be a symptom of dysfunctional uterine bleeding.

Uterine fibroids are a major reason for excessive bleeding.

endometrial hyperplasia

A condition where there is thickening of the uterine lining (overgrowth of cells in the endometrium) that may cause excessive bleeding.

endometrium

The inner lining of the uterus.

endometrial ablation

An outpatient procedure that may involve a laser (or other source) to eliminate the cells lining the uterus. The procedure makes conception impossible.

strual flow. In still other instances there may be a thickening of the uterine lining, a condition called **endometrial hyperplasia**. This thickening is typified by an overgrowth of cells that can lead to abnormal bleeding. Endometrial hyperplasia is another condition that is seen in very young women and those who are nearing menopause. It occurs when estrogen continually stimulates cells of the uterine lining (called the **endometrium**) to divide, causing an overgrowth of cells. Extended estrogen stimulation is not switched off by progesterone (estrogen's chemical antagonist) because progesterone levels are inadequate or missing. While there is no known way to prevent endometrial hyperplasia, your doctor can prescribe progesterone treatment for at least three months to bring the problem under control (see Question #77).

Conservative treatments for abnormal uterine bleeding depend on the bleeding's underlying cause. Treatment may be as simple as a prescription for progesterone-based therapy. However, if you no longer wish to have children, your doctor may suggest a procedure called **endometrial ablation**, which may involve a laser (or other source) to eliminate (ablate) the uterine lining. Endometrial ablation can be performed as an outpatient procedure and you can go home shortly after its completion. You will require little more than Motrin or a similar medication afterward to relieve cramping. Because the procedure destroys the endometrium, fertility may not be possible. Endometrial ablation, which can be performed in several ways, has a very high success rate, although a small percentage of women may still require a hysterectomy. Various ablation techniques are discussed in greater detail in Part 3, along with other uterus-sparing treatments.

While much of this discussion has examined the nature and causes of abnormal uterine bleeding, it is important to take note of the emotional and psychological impact that chronic bleeding can produce. It is not at all unusual to be depressed about any medical condition that can dominate your life. But be advised: Depression itself can become so overwhelming that it, too, evolves into a difficult medical issue in need of attention. The psychological impact of excessive bleeding is said to be a major underreported source of clinical depression in women. Depression is most prevalent in those who have tried a succession of treatments that have provided only intermittent relief.

By addressing the bleeding that has had a negative impact on your quality of life, your depression may be alleviated as well. Of course, it may take awhile for your depression to subside, but the point is to move in the direction of knowing exactly what is affecting you and effectively treating your underlying condition. Additional causes of abnormal uterine bleeding are addressed in Questions #21, #27, #29 and #32, and appropriate treatments are discussed.

17. I am distressed about the persistent pain of endometriosis. Is pain-relief medication a temporary treatment until my physician recommends a hysterectomy?

Simply being treated for pain does not mean that your case automatically will advance to one requiring fertility-ending surgery. Pain relief is an important matter to many (but certainly not all) women affected by endometriosis, a reproductive system disorder in which tissue from the inner lining of the uterus grows in places it should not be. Endometrial tissue implants itself anywhere in the pelvic area: on the ovaries, the bladder, and even the large intestine. These rogue deposits can lead to scar tissue and pain during sexual intercourse and bowel movements. Some patients report a constant dull pain in the abdomen. For many women, the discomfort of endometriosis is extremely intense during menstruation when bouts with cramping can become unbearable.

non-steroidal anti-inflammatory drugs (NSAIDs)

A group of medications (aspirin, ibuprofen, and naproxen) that reduce inflammation and simultaneously affect the natural hormone-like fatty acids known as prostaglandins, which are a major source of pain and inflammation.

prostaglandins

A family of potent hormone-like fatty acids secreted by an array of tissues that can serve as a source of pain and inflammation. Prostaglandins have been implicated in a wide variety of pain syndromes from migraine headaches to uterine cramps.

As will be discussed in Part 5, the condition is exceptionally complex and can strike as young as the teen years. Even though over-the-counter medications can be used to alleviate the discomfort for some women, a health care provider may choose something stronger to address a particularly elevated degree of pain. In your case, your health care provider may choose a prescription-grade drug that belongs to the family of medications known as **non-steroidal anti-inflammatory drugs (NSAIDs)**.

NSAIDs are a very familiar class of drugs and include many well-known and widely used medications. Aspirin, the old medicine cabinet standby, is the original class member, but this group of medications also includes names you may readily recognize: ibuprofen (sold as Motrin and Advil) or naproxen (sold as Aleve and Naprosyn). NSAIDs are important because they reduce inflammation and at the same time act on the natural hormone-like fatty acids in the body known as prostaglandins. **Prostaglandins** are a family of potent compounds that are secreted by an array of tissues and are a major source of pain and inflammation. Prostaglandins have been implicated in a wide variety of pain syndromes from migraine headaches to uterine cramps.

Whether your doctor recommends Indocin (indomethacin) or some other NSAID, the medication is best taken just before your period as well as throughout its duration because of the extreme cramping often associated with endometriosis. Some patients with the condition have constant pain because of the diffuse nature of endometriosis, a matter that may warrant further evaluation and possibly more aggressive treatment, which can include minimally invasive surgery aimed at eliminating renegade endometrial deposits.

NSAIDs work for many patients because they are capable of addressing the two key factors that are at the core of the disorder: pain and inflammation. Other NSAIDs include prescription-grade Motrin, Feldene, Dolobid, and Clinoril, to name a few. Your doctor will want to monitor you closely while you are taking such potent painkillers. Naturally, neither Indocin nor any other NSAID is capable of addressing emotional problems that may have arisen as a result of your endometriosis. Effective pain relief, however, is one way to begin eliminating emotional distress that may have arisen in response to pain, whose intensity some women describe as debilitating.

Still, it cannot be overemphasized that hysterectomy is not the inevitable outcome for patients with endometriosis and actually is considered a treatment of last resort for a majority of patients, even women with the worst symptoms. Because the disorder occurs in young women, many of whom have not had the opportunity to have children, your doctor will work with you to preserve the ability to become pregnant if pregnancy is your goal. Hysterectomy generally enters the discussion only after all other methods of addressing your endometriosis have failed.

18. I have heard that a hysterectomy can cause long-term depression. Is this true?

It is not unusual to be depressed after major surgery of any kind.

It is not unusual to be depressed after major surgery of any kind. While hysterectomy is no exception, by itself it cannot induce a complex psychological condition that persists for months or possibly even years after the surgery. Research—including a landmark study—has proven this point. Immediately after a hysterectomy, especially an abdominal procedure, many patients are not as mobile as they would like to be. There are rules the doctor has imposed regarding bathing, sex, and exercise. Patients are out of work for a month or more recuperating. It is easy enough to grasp how this temporary change can induce a mild depression. Nevertheless, studies show that the majority of women bounce back after their operations once they have resumed their usual daily routines.

While there has been much discussion over the Internet about hysterectomies triggering depression, many women have found that depression that existed prior to surgery subsided once they were free of the disorder that led to hysterectomy. Being free of persistent pain, bleeding, or both eliminates a psychological burden. A study of nearly 1,300 patients who underwent hysterectomies for pelvic pain concluded that women who suffered from depression at the time of their surgeries experienced improvements in their depression, quality of life, and sexual function after having a hysterectomy. These scientific findings are in no way a recommendation for the surgery, but are mentioned here to help put into context how some women fared psychologically after their operations.

The University of North Carolina researchers, reporting in the journal *Obstetrics and Gynecology*, noted that depression is the most common disorder known to accompany pelvic pain. Their research, which was led by Dr. Katherine Hartmann (director of the University of North Carolina's Center for Women's Health Research), is considered a landmark because it answered a question that had persisted for decades: Does hysterectomy cause depression? Results, at least from this study, suggest that the answer is a resounding "no!"

Even so, a single study does not provide an answer for every situation, especially when it comes to a surgery as pervasive as hysterectomy. Smaller studies have turned up a range of different results that you may want to consider. For example, research has shown that women who experience long-term depression after a hysterectomy are often those who experienced serious depression before their operations, and usually for reasons other than the abnormal bleeding or pain that led to a hysterectomy.

Further studies have demonstrated that women who experience a hysterectomy-related side effect (such as a post-operative infection that requires additional treatment, hospitalization, and possibly a longer recovery) are likely to develop post-surgical depression. Statistics from the CDC indicate the likelihood of post-operative infection is low but that the risk is 1.7 times higher following an abdominal hysterectomy. Another group likely to develop depression is composed of women who quickly chose to have the surgery without first weighing their options about alternatives. An end to childbearing capability may be difficult to accept, especially if the woman believed she was forced into the surgery, had little time to think about it, and regretted the decision afterward.

If you suspect that you may be vulnerable to depression, it may be helpful to try to recognize some of its symptoms and to discuss them with your physician. Even though it is a mental condition, **depression** (an unshakeable sense of sadness, dejection, and hopelessness) can have physical effects, mental health experts say. People who are clinically depressed often find they are experiencing changes in their sleep patterns; either they are sleeping longer or sleeping less. Many people who are depressed experience inexplicable aches and pains. True depression often is accompanied by an overwhelming sense of fatigue and a loss of interest in sex, hobbies, and even people who once were a source of joy. Two important hallmarks of the disorder are feelings of hopelessness and helplessness. If you experience these symptoms before or after a hysterectomy, it is very important to talk to your doctor, who will be able to help you get the care you need.

depression

A mental condition marked by sadness, inactivity, and an inability to think clearly. Depression is also characterized by feelings of dejection or hopelessness, and a significant increase or decrease in sleeping. In severe cases there may be suicidal tendencies.

19. Can my gynecologist treat depression?

Gynecologists are very familiar with the depression that occurs as a result of excessive pain and bleeding. They know that these conditions affect you psychologically, possibly as much as they do physically. Your gynecologist will probably talk to you about depression and let you know that having any type of chronic medical condition can have a strong impact on your quality of life, your ability to go about your day-to-day tasks, and efforts to maintain your role in the lives of those who depend on you, such as your children, your spouse, partner, or elderly parents.

Your gynecologist certainly will talk to you within the context of what women with similar degrees of pain or bleeding experience and how they have coped with these medical conditions. If your depression is particularly deep and your moods so dark that you are having difficulty coping with life—let alone your problem with abnormal pain or bleeding—then your gynecologist probably will recommend that you see a mental health expert such as a licensed social worker (LCSW or MSW), a licensed clinical psychologist (PhD), or psychiatrist (MD), who can help you put matters into perspective and, at the same time, begin therapy for your depression. It is not unusual for women who are being treated for a reproductive system disorder to be simultaneously treated for depression. In addition to counseling, you may also be prescribed an antidepressant if it is determined that medication will best address your mental state.

20. I am totally stressed over my "female" problems. I feel frightened about the excessive bleeding and clotting during lengthy menstrual periods. Will reducing my stress eliminate the abnormal bleeding?

It is normal to feel that stress is increasing the amount of your bleeding, but actually things may be the other way around. Excessive bleeding, especially when it presents with excessive clotting or other symptoms, may exacerbate the amount of stress you feel. It may be scary to see exceptional amounts of blood.

Of course, this is not to diminish the impact that stress can have in your life. Stress is very difficult to cope with no matter what the source, especially today when it may be compounded by demands of a career, family, and commitments associated with a busy life. Each of these might contribute to the amount of pressure you are feeling. Stress can raise levels of certain "fight or flight" hormones, like adrenaline, that increase your heart rate and blood pressure, and escalate your level of anxiety. Many women report that their bleeding and cramping increase when their levels of stress are high.

Are you under pressure at work? Do you have financial concerns? Have your medical bills outstripped your ability to pay? Has your medical condition strained a personal relationship? Your first impulse with respect to your reproductive organs may be, "Just rip them out." Stop. Take a deep breath. Count to 10 while slowly exhaling (or 20, which ever works best), and realize that there are other solutions. Be honest with your physician and lay out your concerns about abnormal uterine bleeding as well as your level of stress.

It is very likely that once your health care provider dis-covers the source of your excessive bleeding and has prescribed effective treatment, your level of stress will subside. But just so you fully understand that a hys-terectomy is not recommended as a first-choice proce-dure, you also should feel assured that you are probably not facing an imminent surgery and weeks of recovery, so that is one stress-producing issue you can cast aside. There are steps that can be taken to put virtually all of your issues involving stress into perspective.

Gynecologists throughout the United States have long been aware that stress is an important and damaging component of any abnormal bleeding or pain-producing pelvic condition. Your doctor may recommend stress management sessions overseen by a therapist. Your local medical center may be one of a growing number that offers complementary medical techniques, or can direct you to centers that provide such services. These forms of therapy might include exercise classes, relaxation, or massage therapies. If you tend more toward something with a New Age spin, perhaps guided imagery, aroma, or chroma therapies may help reduce your level of stress. While they are unconventional, you may find that any one or a combination of them won't hurt, and they actually might help.

21. I have been diagnosed with anemia. Is that the cause of my emotional distress and depression? Would a hysterectomy solve my problem with anemia?

Anemia does not cause depression but it can, as mentioned earlier, lead to extreme exhaustion. When your cells are deprived of oxygen, you are anemic. It may seem to you that extraordinary amounts of energy must be summoned to complete simple day-to-day tasks. When you have anemia, just getting out of bed in the morning and going about your routine may seem laborious and tiresome.

Depression, however, is a different matter altogether because it may be the reason you lose interest in activities you once enjoyed or the reason you find yourself crying for no apparent reason. Just as abnormal uterine bleeding is a reason to avoid going out with friends, shunning sex, or calling in sick to work, so it is with depression. Both anemia and depression have a way of sapping your strength and your *joie de vivre*. Certainly, this does not mean that a hysterectomy must be performed. Your health care provider will want to address both the underlying problem that is causing your abnormal bleeding and the anemia, which if it worsens, can prove life threatening.

A normal blood hemoglobin reading for a healthy woman is about 15 grams. Hemoglobin is the molecule in red blood cells that carries oxygen. For those with significant anemia caused by abnormal uterine bleeding, however, the hemoglobin reading may drop as low as 5, a level that is so low that patients must be hospitalized. Some women must be treated in emergency rooms because of low blood oxygen. Anemia can be treated. In unusual cases when the hemoglobin level is desperately low, blood transfusions may be in order. When the anemia is milder, your doctor probably will recommend dietary iron supplementation. To treat it correctly, as mentioned earlier, the underlying uterine disorder that caused excessive bleeding in the first place must be addressed.

You can think about anemia, abnormal uterine bleeding, and depression as having a domino effect. Abnormal uterine bleeding causes anemia, which in turn causes extreme exhaustion, which amplifies the emotional distress and depression that has occurred because of continuous blood loss. Anemia is a serious side effect of abnormal uterine bleeding because when it is extreme, it not only can cause fainting, it can be life threatening.

If you have uterine fibroids, which are often associated with serious abnormal bleeding, you may be a candidate for a procedure that allows your doctor to eliminate the blood supply to your fibroids (see Question #51). In this procedure, fibroids are forced to shrink and you have the added benefit of a uterus that is left intact. Once fibroids are no longer causing blood loss, your blood hemoglobin levels can return to a normal level.

22. I am 22 years old and have had excessive menstrual bleeding and cramping for two years. My mother says I will probably have to have a hysterectomy like other women in my family. I am very hesitant about seeing a gynecologist. What options do I have?

It is important that you see a gynecologist about abnormal bleeding. Lengthy periods and abdominal cramping can occur for a variety of reasons at your age. Just because your relatives have had hysterectomies does not mean that you must have one, too. Hysterectomy is not a first choice therapy. You have to ask yourself two key questions: Can I go on living with excessive bleeding and cramping? Have I explored all of my options?

Menorrhagia (mentioned briefly in Question #16) simply means excessive menstrual bleeding. A key characteristic of menorrhagia is that it occurs at the regular time of the menstrual cycle; it generally refers to menstrual periods that last longer than seven days and require in excess of 10 pads per day. For some women, a menstrual period might run even longer, lasting nonstop up to 12 days, and requires even more padding. Cramping and/or more prolonged pain along with severe clotting are typical symptoms of the condition for still other women. About 20% of young women experience heavy menstrual bleeding that can interfere

About 20% of young women experience heavy menstrual bleeding that can interfere with their quality of life.

with their quality of life. It is important to understand your menstrual cycles and how they are affecting your general sense of health.

Normally, a menstrual cycle runs every 28 days, but that is not a hard and fast rule that describes everyone's cycle. For some women, the cycle can range between every 21 to every 35 days. Those ranges are still considered normal. Interestingly, menorrhagia can have any one of several underlying causes: hormone imbalances, fibroids, **endometrial polyps** (small benign growths that protrude into the uterus), endometriosis, intrauterine devices used for birth control, hypothyroidism, and even autoimmune disorders, such as lupus. Your physician is trained to differentiate among all of these causes.

With respect to a hormonal imbalance, menstrual cycles may be characterized by too much estrogen or perhaps too little progesterone. Inadequate progesterone levels fail to counterbalance the effects of estrogen, which means that the second half of your menstrual cycle (where the hormone progesterone is released to slow down and halt the flow of blood) does not counteract estrogen's effects. Sufferers may experience light bleeding between periods and especially heavy bleeding while diagnoses.

Doctors learned long ago, after performing hysterectomies on some women who experienced excessive menstrual bleeding, that the uterus was free of any underlying condition! The uterus that had been removed was completely healthy, which means there was no sound medical reason for a hysterectomy. Talk to your physician about your symptoms and discuss ways in which abnormal bleeding is treated without resorting to invasive surgery. This is especially impor-

endometrial polyps

Small benign growths that protrude into the uterus.

tant in your case because you are a young woman and have not yet had children. You have options.

Perhaps your gynecologist can prescribe medication to relieve the bleeding. Birth control pills may achieve this by regulating your menstrual cycles. Moreover, hysterectomy very rarely is used as a treatment for abnormal bleeding in younger women. Do not rely on faulty wisdom or family experiences when it comes to your health. You need a proper diagnosis from a gynecologist who can evaluate your problem and recommend appropriate treatment. Freeing yourself from what you believe is a family legacy of hysterectomies may be your most effective step toward alleviating depression.

You may even want to ask yourself why your relatives had hysterectomies. Were they affected by abnormal menstrual cycles? Did they experience constant abdominal pain? Those two symptoms could point to different underlying reproductive system conditions. You also might want to consider this mind-boggling possibility: It is very likely that they may not have had the same medical condition that you have. For that matter, they may not have even had a medical condition. A generation ago, unscrupulous doctors performed hysterectomies for flimsy medical reasons. It is because of those practices that women's health advocacy remains so strong today.

If you don't get good answers from the first doctor you see, try visiting another for a second opinion, or even a third or fourth. Don't stop seeking a solution until you get valid answers. You should want to take whatever steps necessary to fully understand why you are experiencing bleeding and cramping, and as a result, suffering substantial emotional distress and depression.

23. I am 55 and have been spotting recently. I am an emotional wreck because of this. Could this be residual menstrual cycles? I stopped menstruating three years ago.

There is no recognized medical condition called a "residual menstrual cycle" that occurs after you have become post-menopausal. Additionally, it would be difficult for your physician even to tell you what the source of the bleeding is without a thorough examination. Bleeding after menopause could be a sign of a serious problem that needs to be evaluated by your health care provider, and the sooner the better. Of course, it is understandable that you are emotionally distressed about abnormal bleeding. But it is very important to bear in mind that post-menopausal bleeding can be a harbinger of bad news. There is no time for dawdling, guessing, or self-diagnosing. Once your periods end, they end for good and do not show up two, three or ten years later. Bleeding after menopause is not a sign that you have somehow signed a new lease on youth.

Endometrial cancer is the most common gynecologic malignancy in the United States and its incidence increases with age. Its earliest symptom is vaginal bleeding that usually occurs after menopause. The disease is extraordinarily rare in young women from their mid teens through their late 20s, but the number of cases rise with each increasing decade, reaching a peak incidence among women between the ages of 60 and 70. Bleeding after menopause is almost always a serious matter unless you are taking hormone replacement therapy (HRT), during which time menstrual-like bleeding and spotting can occur. But spotting at age 55 in a woman not taking HRT pills courts danger each day gone by without seeing a doctor.

In addition to endometrial cancer, abnormal bleeding at this age might be a symptom of any other form of cancer, such as ovarian, cervical, or a rare reproductive system tumor. Conditions that affect younger women, such as fibroids, menorrhagia, and the uterine disorder known as adenomyosis, also associated with abnormal bleeding, are no longer part of an older woman's reality. There is no way for any individual to diagnose the source of her own bleeding, nor would it be smart to summarily dismiss it as "not important" or benign.

The first rule of thumb when dealing with post-menopausal bleeding is to make an appointment for a full examination, preferably from a gynecologist. Moving quickly not only helps to resolve the bleeding, taking action might save your life. Thinking that the problem will go away on its own certainly is unwise. Waiting may only allow the matter to worsen, and thus transform something treatable into a serious and possibly deadly condition. If cancer is confirmed, you may be facing a hysterectomy. The aim of the surgery for women with cancer is to remove the tumor and affected tissue from your body.

PART THREE

Understanding How Healthy Reproductive Organs Function

What are the organs that make up the female reproductive system? Why is the uterus so important?

How do estrogen and progesterone differ?

What causes perimenopause and menopause?

More . . .

24. What are the organs that make up the female reproductive system? Why is the uterus so important?

The female reproductive organs consist of five principal structures: the vagina, the cervix, the uterus, a pair of fallopian tubes, and two ovaries. The **vagina** is the passageway from the outside of the body to the reproductive system's interior. Located at the other end of the vagina, proceeding into the body, is the **cervix**. It is the narrow opening into the uterus. The **uterus** (womb) is a pear-shaped hollow organ about three inches long and two inches wide at its top. Even though the uterus is hollow, it is a very dynamic organ. It plays a role in the monthly menstrual cycle, provides an environment for the growth and nourishment of a developing fetus and produces mild contractile waves as part of the female sexual response.

Think of this organ's interior as having the shape of an inverted triangle, and it is from this cavity that the lining (called the endometrium) is shed monthly as menstrual flow. Menstruation occurs because each month the endometrium thickens to prepare the uterus for pregnancy. When pregnancy does not occur, the endometrium breaks down and is released from the body. In instances when a pregnancy is established, the endometrium then accepts and protects the fertilized egg.

The uterus is an extraordinarily elastic organ. Composed of smooth muscle, it is capable of stretching several times its normal size to accommodate a full-term pregnancy. Imagine its elasticity among women who have carried quadruplets, quintuplets, and even septuplets to term. But just as a uterus is able to stretch to accommodate a pregnancy of multiples, it also is capa-

vagina
The passageway from the outside of the body to the reproductive system's interior.

cervix
The neck at the lower end of the uterus. It connects the uterus to the vagina. The cervix dilates during labor to allow the birth of a baby.

uterus
Also called the womb; a pear-shaped hollow organ about three inches long and two inches wide at its top; has a role in the monthly menstrual cycle, provides an environment for the growth and nourishment of a developing fetus, and produces mild contractile waves as part of the female sexual response.

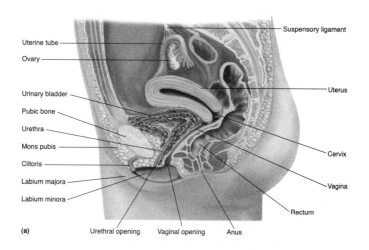

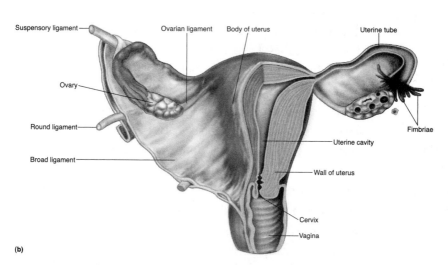

The female reproductive system. (a) Midsagittal section. (b) Anterior view.

ble of stretching several times its size to accommodate the growth of fibroid tumors, some of which have the capacity to reach the size of a full term pregnancy and even larger. Another disorder, uterine prolapse, is marked by the uterus's loss of positioning in the pelvic area. The organ can bulge into the vagina, a condition that necessitates a hysterectomy. You may find it interesting to note that the uterus is anchored with eight ligaments. In a hysterectomy, whether it is performed abdominally or vaginally, these eight ligaments are cut to free the organ from the body.

25. What is the role of the two fallopian tubes?

fallopian tubes

Also known as the oviducts; located at the top part of the uterus (the fundus), they are the conduits through which eggs cells (ova) are transported to the uterus. At their uppermost ends, the tubes have fingerlike projections that sweep eggs from the ovaries. Each tube measures about four inches in length and possesses contractile capability, a motion that allows them to propel an egg into the uterus.

The **fallopian tubes**, also known as the oviducts, are attached to the top part of the uterus (the fundus) and serve as the conduits through which eggs cells (ova) are transported to the uterus. At their uppermost ends, the tubes are characterized by fingerlike projections whose role is to sweep eggs from the ovaries into the tubes. Each tube measures about four inches in length. The fallopian tubes have contractile capability, the motion that allows them to propel an egg into the uterus. When an egg is not fertilized, it breaks apart and is cast away with menstrual flow. In instances when the fertilized egg does not properly travel into the uterus and becomes lodged in a fallopian tube, a tubal pregnancy can result. Known medically as an ectopic pregnancy, this situation may prove life threatening for the mother. It is often discovered at the point of an emergency when the woman is experiencing severe abdominal pain. An ectopic pregnancy necessitates the surgical removal of the affected fallopian tube. It is not always necessary to remove the fallopian tubes during a hysterectomy and in some cases they are left intact.

26. Why are the ovaries so important?

Pulitzer Prize winning author Natalie Angier, in her book *Female Geography*, wrote that up close and personal the ovaries look like two clumps of oatmeal. At first this may sound like a rather unseemly way of describing the very structures that help orchestrate the flow of female hormones and provide the eggs to begin a new life. But though not pretty, the **ovaries** are two of the most dynamic structures in the body.

In fact, the very lumpiness of these structures is a result of the eruption of eggs, which leaves the ovarian surface uneven. Each month one or the other ovary releases a single egg from a follicle that has developed deep within it. This process usually occurs midway, around day 14, of a 28-day ovulation cycle.

These twin structures are located on either side of the uterus. Each contains thousands of eggs, or ova (also known as germ cells because they are capable of germinating when fertilized). One egg is released per month starting at puberty and continuing in this clocklike pattern throughout most of the reproductive years.

In terms of size, the two oval-shaped glands are about that of an almond in women of reproductive age, though they are considerably smaller in those who are past menopause.

Chemically, estrogen and progesterone are two key products of these glands. These hormones will be discussed in greater detail in Questions #14 and #27. Estrogen causes the thickening of the endometrium and the vagina each month in the earliest phase of the menstrual cycle. Progesterone is the primary hormone that influences menstruation and maintains pregnancy. As a woman gets closer to menopause, she often produces no eggs and less and less of the ovarian hormones. Gradually, usually in her early 50s (in the United States, the average age for menopause is 51), menstrual periods cease.

ovary
Twin oval-shaped glands about the size of an almond, located on either side of the uterus, that contain thousands of ova (also known as germ cells). One egg is released per month, starting at puberty and continuing in a clocklike pattern throughout most of the reproductive years.

The ovaries are two of the most dynamic structures in the body.

27. How do estrogen and progesterone differ?

These two compounds are the principle female sex hormones that are responsible for a wide range of vital chemical activities. Each also carries out important functions during pregnancy; their concentration (too little of one or the other) also play roles in certain reproductive system disorders. The two hormones have several similarities, but each has chemical functions that make it distinctly different. For example, both are steroid hormones secreted by the ovaries. These two hormones are vital to menstruation and are timed to perform their specific chemical tasks during different critical phases of the cycle.

Of the two, estrogen plays a dominant role in an array of biological functions. During puberty, the hormone triggers the development of so-called secondary sex characteristics, such as development of the breasts, pubic hair and female vocal timbre. Estrogen also has other important activities. It is known to protect the integrity of the skeletal system and thwart the development of cardiovascular disease by helping to maintain the elasticity of blood vessels. It also helps maintain normal brain function and muscle tone.

follicle-stimulating hormone (FSH)

Produced by the pituitary gland in the brain; when suppressed by estrogen, FSH inhibits ovulation in the earlier phase of the menstrual cycle.

One of estrogen's primary roles is suppressing **follicle-stimulating hormone (FSH)**, which is produced by the pituitary gland in the brain. By suppressing FSH, ovulation in the earlier phase of the menstrual cycle is stopped while estrogen goes about its work, thickening the endometrium.

FSH is a gonadotropic hormone, meaning that it stimulates the ovaries and is essential for reproduction. FSH is released or suppressed by sex hormones in a complex action known as a negative feedback loop at various stages of the menstrual cycle.

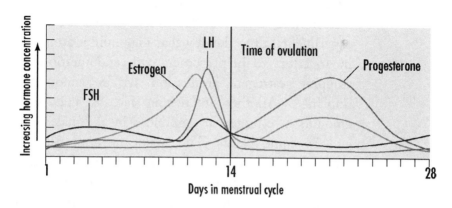

Changes in relative concentrations of hormones during ovulation and menstruation.

Borrowing an idea from nature, medical scientists were able to make oral contraceptives based on that same principle. They developed synthetic estrogenic compounds to inhibit FSH. Without ovulation, pregnancy cannot occur. Synthetic estrogen also is used in estrogen replacement therapy to abate the effects of menopausal symptoms. A synthetic estrogen medication such as Premarin might be chosen after a hysterectomy and oophorectomy to treat hot flashes and other disquieting symptoms. Estrogen is secreted in the first half of the ovulatory cycle and is involved in thickening the uterus and vagina.

You may find it interesting to note that estrogen is produced in abundance in pre-menopausal women by the ovaries and, to a lesser extent, by the adrenal glands (located on top of both kidneys), which produce androgen hormones that are converted to estrogen. In post-menopausal women, androgen hormone conversion is the primary source of estrogen after the decline of ovarian hormone production. The conversion of androgens into estrogen is known to occur in several types of tissue, but particularly fat cells. An enzyme by the name of aromatase catalyzes the conversion (see Question #59 for a discussion on an experimental drug therapy that may inhibit aromatase in an effort to help women with endometriosis by stopping estrogen production within endometrial implants). Another interesting fact is that small amounts of estrogen are produced by the male testes and by some plants. The major form of estrogen secreted by the ovaries is known as estradiol, which is converted to estrone in the bloodstream. During pregnancy, the primary form of estrogen is estradiol, which is produced by the placenta. In all, these three forms of the hormone produce estrogenic activity in humans.

As beneficial as estrogen may be, its presence can underlie several major female reproductive conditions. Its secretion has been linked to the growth of fibroid tumors, which can gain bulk under estrogen's influence and lead to abnormal uterine bleeding, miscarriages, and infertility in some cases. Endometriosis is another condition influenced by estrogen. The disorder is typified by rogue deposits of endometrial tissue that proliferate outside of the uterus, causing pain, irregular menstrual bleeding, and in the worst of cases, scarring and infertility. Estrogen also can serve as the chemical fuel that drives the growth of certain gynecologic cancers.

Progesterone, on the other hand, can be seen as estrogen's antagonist. It is produced during the luteal phase (or second two weeks of the menstrual cycle) and is important because it prepares the endometrium (the tissue lining the uterus) for the implantation of a fertilized egg. It is progesterone that influences the shedding of the endometrium as menstrual flow when a pregnancy does not occur. Menstruation is triggered because progesterone levels fall when a fertilized egg is not present. Progesterone is not released into the bloodstream as a constant flow but enters the blood in spurts. As a result, its levels are not always consistent. However, during pregnancy, progesterone levels remain stable because the hormone is needed to maintain the pregnancy. During this time, the hormone is no longer produced by the ovaries but by the placenta. When the baby is delivered, progesterone levels fall, which spurs the process of lactation. Like estrogen, progesterone is a steroid hormone, which means that at a molecular level it consists of four connected ring structures and is synthesized in the body from a derivative of cholesterol.

Progesterone therapy has become important in the treatment of several reproductive system disorders, including endometriosis. Synthetic versions of the hormone are known as progestins, which are useful in hormone replacement therapy for women with a uterus because they protect the endometrium from developing cancer. During perimenopause (the period of time immediately before menopause), progesterone levels are the first to decline. As a result of this loss, progesterone levels are very low in post-menopausal women.

28. What causes perimenopause and menopause?

The cyclic activity of estrogen and progesterone declines with age, leading to the cessation of menstrual periods in middle age. The diminishing presence of the body's principal female hormones is neither abrupt nor comes as a surprise, because women usually in their mid-40s, notice that their menstrual cycle begins to change perceptibly. This transitional stage is known as peri-menopause and is a noteworthy period of life for a variety of reasons. Not only does this transitional period serve as a prelude to menopause and an end to fertility, it is also a time when certain medical conditions become more prevalent. There is a decrease in bone density because of a declining estrogen supply, and this may cause **osteopenia** to be a concern for some women. Although bone density has decreased, there is not always an increased risk for fracture.

osteopenia

A condition of decreased calcification or density of bone.

Certainly, there are changes in the menstrual cycle itself, such as the absence of ovulation, as women get closer to menopause. This explains fertility problems among women in their 40s when they attempt to conceive. Fertilization cannot occur when the ovaries have only a paltry few (if any) eggs left to release. The peri-menopause years can be marked by heavy menstrual flow as a result of the menstrual cycle lingering in the estrogen phase. Some women experience erratic cycles from one month to the next because the cyclic familiarity to which they had become so accustomed over decades of menstruating is lost due to fluctuating hormone levels. Estrogen and progesterone are no longer produced in the pattern that marked their flow for so many years.

The simple truth about perimenopause is that the ovaries are going out of the egg production business for good and they are throwing the menstrual cycle, for many women, into hormonal turmoil. Some months may be characterized by clotting; others may be note-worthy because a period doesn't come at all, giving the false impression that menopause has occurred. Women soon learn that perimenopause is full of surprises because a period, or at least what now has to be defined as one, may resume after a respite of 48 days or more. The follicles are producing eggs only now and then, so there is no follicular remnant (i.e., *corpus luteum*) from which progesterone can be secreted. The result is a lack of a consistent presence of progesterone to work as it once had, regulating the menstrual cycle. It should come as no surprise that between the two major ovarian hormones progesterone is the first to go.

Menopause, meanwhile, is the point in a woman's life when menstruation forever ceases, usually in the early 50s, though sometimes earlier (and in some cases later). The strictest definition of menopause is a cessation of menstrual cycles for one year, the period after which is known as post-menopause. Although menopause is a natural part of aging, it also can be induced surgically when the ovaries of a pre-menopausal woman are removed in a bilateral oophorectomy.

PART FOUR

Reproductive Organ Disorders: Fibroids

What are uterine fibroids?

Why are fibroids called tumors? Can they become cancerous?

Why do women develop fibroids?

More . . .

29. What are uterine fibroids?

Uterine fibroids are benign tumors that develop within the cavity of the uterus, on its surface, or between its walls, and are the single most common reason for hysterectomies in the United States. An estimated 200,000 hysterectomies are performed nationwide each year because of fibroid tumors. Nearly 30% of all hysterectomies are performed because of these growths. Fibroids are the most common non-cancerous tumor in women of reproductive age and are the source of a broad spectrum of pelvic problems, which range from chronic pain to excessive, frequent, and unpredictable uterine bleeding.

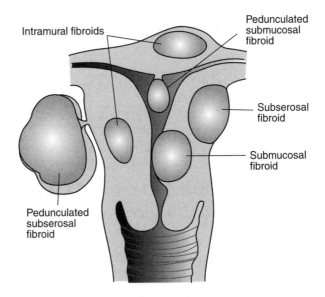

Known interchangeably as a fibromyoma, leiomyoma, or just plain old myoma, a fibroid can vary from the size of a pea to that of a grapefruit. Decades ago, when women were less likely to seek immediate medical attention for pelvic disorders, doctors frequently saw fibroids that were the size of full-term pregnancies.

Such growths rarely are seen today but are still known to occur. It is still common in the United States to diagnose fibroids that are of a significant enough size to cause the abdomen to protrude. The largest fibroid ever removed is reported to have weighed an astounding 140 pounds! You may find it surprising when your gynecologist first conveys the size of your fibroid in terms of a growing fetus. Your doctor may tell you that your fibroid is the size of a twelve-, thirteen- or fourteen-week pregnancy.

Because fibroids can grow anywhere in the uterus and in a wide range of sizes, they are associated with a variety of uterine problems. The growths are most notable for triggering heavy menstrual bleeding, disabling cramps, and unpredictable bleeding between periods, and may underlie serious anemia and exhaustion resulting from blood loss. An estimated 30% of women with fibroids experience abnormal uterine bleeding that usually does not begin as extreme blood loss. For most, the build-up to very heavy periods occurs gradually over many months until the flow is persistent and, in some cases, life-threatening when blood loss leads to severe anemia. Some women with fibroids report they never seem to stop menstruating, that one period seems to flow into the next. In some instances, large clots may occur along with the bleeding. As fibroids continue to grow, so do the problems. Additional concerns include miscarriages and infertility.

Patients also report feelings of "fullness" in the pelvic area, a condition medically referred to as **pelvic pressure**. The benign tumors also can cause hemorrhoids because of fibroid-induced pressure on the anus. Fecal incontinence may affect some women while constipation is a problem of others. Urinary incontinence affects

pelvic pressure

A sensation of "fullness" in the abdomen; can be caused by fibroids.

still other women because of fibroid pressure on the bladder. The pressure can become so problematic that women are forced to wear padding to prevent embarrassment. If you are experiencing any of these symptoms, you should report them to your gynecologist and undergo a full work-up for your symptoms.

Scientists at the National Institutes of Health estimate that anywhere from 50% to 80% of women will develop one or more fibroid tumors by the time they reach their 35th birthday. Curiously, when all of the troublesome symptoms are taken into account, only 25% of patients diagnosed with fibroids experience problems serious enough to seek medical treatment. Just as fibroids may prove to be painful nuisances in some women, they are painless and quiescent in others, and their presence is known only after they are discovered during a routine pelvic examination. Indeed, a majority of women with fibroids never report adverse symptoms.

Guidelines from the American College of Obstetrics and Gynecology strongly emphasize that treatment of uterine fibroids should be avoided unless the growths are producing symptoms that interfere with the quality of life. While it is prudent to get a proper diagnosis of your fibroid (or fibroids because some women have more than one), you should not expect to undergo treatment unless the condition is causing abnormal uterine bleeding, severe pain, miscarriages, interference with conception, or incontinence (fecal or urinary). Medical scientists have developed several alternative treatments to hysterectomy for women with problematic fibroid tumors, which will be discussed in greater detail elsewhere in this section. You may find it interesting to note that despite a growing amount of study devoted to fibroid tumors by medical scientists around the world, the growths still pose numerous research questions and a host of medical mysteries.

30. Why are fibroids called tumors? Can they become cancerous?

Although fibroids are called tumors, these growths are composed of harmless cells. When they reach sufficient enough size, fibroids can put pressure on other organs, or distort the shape of the uterus. Decades of studies have demonstrated that it is extraordinarily rare for a fibroid to become cancerous. Those that do, however, develop into the type of malignancy known as a **sarcoma**. They are so unusual that U.S. health statistics show they occur in fewer than 1% of women who are diagnosed with the growths. Fibroids tend to shrink with age and become progressively less bothersome with time.

sarcoma

A highly malignant type of tumor; connective tissue neoplasm.

Still, fibroids can grow in unwieldy ways, sometimes even on a stalk called a pedicle, in which case they are known as **pedunculated fibroids**. These fibroids usually grow on the outside of the uterus. No matter how or where they grow, fibroids can obstruct and sometimes even seriously impair the function of healthy uterine tissue, leading to physical problems and emotional anxieties for many women. Even though these fibroids are abnormal, the cells from which they are derived are not life-threatening. In other words, the fibroid cells, unlike cancerous cells, are compatible with life.

pedunculated fibroids

A type of fibroid that grows on a stalk usually on the outside of the uterus.

Fibroids tend to shrink with age and become progressively less bothersome with time.

A key feature of fibroids is their tendency to develop in knotty bundles. Up close, these bundles that comprise the inner tissue of a fibroid appear as compacted swirls. There are other structural components, such as collagen and proteins, which help give fibroid tumors their characteristic look and shape. The very name "fibroid" is derived from the fact that the growths are mostly made of fibrous tissue. Fibroids are capable of growing to various sizes inside and on the outside of the uterus, and occasionally even on other pelvic structures that are made of smooth muscle. Because fibroid tumors are capable of gaining bulk and size as a result of exposure to estrogen coursing through the blood, it should come as no surprise that the growths become problematic during peak childbearing years.

31. Why do women develop fibroids?

Very little is known about the cause of uterine fibroid tumors, although scientists have advanced several provocative theories. Unfortunately, none fully explains why fibroids develop, let alone why some remain harmless and others become such renegades and are sources of both physical and emotional pain. Recent studies have suggested that hormones, the environment, and genetics may play individual roles or act in combination as underlying causes. No one knows for sure. Clinicians have long recognized that fibroid growth is intimately linked with the secretion of estrogen. When women reach menopause and ovarian hormone production declines, fibroids tend to shrink dramatically, and in many women they even disappear. But some scientists contend that the estrogen link may be more associated with the growth of fibroids as opposed to what makes them develop in the first place. While some experts have said the tumors tend to grow in women who produce higher than normal levels of estrogen, laboratory tests have shown that some women whose estrogen secretion is clearly within normal ranges also develop the growths.

Scientists are vigorously searching for clues about the origin, growth, and ultimate shrinkage of fibroid tumors. If enough clues are found, medical scientists believe they will be able to piece together a sketchy outline of the natural history of fibroid tumors. Already, at least one prominent clue has surfaced. It involves recent discoveries about certain proteins found in fibroid cells. These discoveries ultimately may help scientists unveil further information on how fibroids seed themselves in the uterus and then grow under the influence of estrogen. Researchers in the reproductive endocrinology division of the National Institutes of Health (Bethesda, MD) have found that fibroids have very low levels of a key structural protein that helps hold normal tissue in place. The protein is called **dermatopontin** and it is a major chemical component your body makes to prevent cells from straying into aberrant patterns of growth. In a healthy uterus, adequate supplies of dermatopontin help maintain the integrity of the organ by keeping uterine cells where they are supposed to be.

dermatopontin

A protein made by the body to prevent cells from straying into aberrant patterns of growth. Researchers have associated low levels of the protein with the development of fibroid tumors.

Fibroids and similar benign growths (such as keloids, which are a type of thick tissue that forms after an incision or wound) tend to have low levels of dermatopontin. A lack of sufficient supplies of the protein may explain why a small portion of the uterus inexplicably develops a fibrous nodule that, over time, can grow and grow until it reaches the size of a golf ball or even a cantaloupe and becomes known as a fibroid tumor. If you were to view fibroid tissue under the microscope, you would notice that its very low levels of dermatopontin cause the tumors to have very disorganized and unstructured strands of collagen. Aside from that feature and the very fact that fibroids tend to have low levels of dermatopontin, scientists have yet to discover other roles that the protein may have in the uterus. Studies of this important chemical component in uterine cells, however, are continuing.

Meanwhile, scientists at the National Institute of Environmental Health Sciences (Research Triangle Park, NC) have been researching whether chemical compounds in the environment, mostly pesticides, are capable of mimicking estrogen. If they do so, scientists are asking whether these chemicals are linked to the development of fibroids and other reproductive system disorders, such as endometriosis. Estrogen-like compounds are common in the environment. Some scientists have theorized that these chemicals compete with your body's natural estrogen for sites on your cells known as "estrogen receptors." It is theorized, but not yet proven, that once a fake estrogen molecule latches onto an estrogen receptor, it can not only block natural estrogen, but it may also unlock the cell and serve as the fuel that drives its growth. The result, the theory holds, may be abnormal growth, such as what your doctor detects in the case of fibroids and other female reproductive system disorders.

In terms of a hereditary link to fibroids, doctors also have long known that women with first-degree relatives (mothers and sisters) diagnosed with the growths are more likely to have fibroids themselves. Problematic fibroids are often seen among relatives, and this observation has had an influence on hysterectomies that have occurred over multiple generations in families. As was underscored in Part 1, many American women may feel the necessity to have a hysterectomy based on their mother's experience, or the experience of another close female relative. Scientists at NIH estimate that while vast numbers of women develop uterine fibroid tumors, about 75% of patients who are diagnosed with them never experience symptoms.

32. Why do fibroids cause abnormal uterine bleeding?

More than any other fibroid-related complaint, abnormal uterine bleeding is the reason most women visit their doctors. Abnormal uterine bleeding also is the underlying reason many women with fibroid tumors choose to have hysterectomies. Excessive bleeding may be linked to one of the least common type of fibroids, called a submucous or submucosal fibroid. Regardless of the term, they refer to the same type of growth. This kind of fibroid tumor develops directly beneath the surface of the endometrium, the inner lining of the uterus. Even though submucosal fibroids may not be as common as their cousin fibroids that grow in other parts of the uterus, they are the cause of the most trouble.

Submucosal fibroids not only are associated with abnormal uterine bleeding, they also have been linked to miscarriages and complications of pregnancy. If you are anemic, have experienced several months of prolonged menstrual bleeding, and are known to have fibroids, a submucosal fibroid may be the type of fibroid (or fibroids) that you have. Of course, your physician will extensively evaluate you before arriving at this diagnosis because there are other causes of uterine bleeding. When your physician examines you for the possible presence of a submucosal fibroid, she or he also will want to rule out any other possible cause of abnormal bleeding, such as ovarian or colorectal cancer. In addition to a manual pelvic examination, your doctor will want a biopsy of your endometrial tissue. A **biopsy** is a procedure in which a tiny sample of uterine tissue is removed so that the cells can be viewed under a microscope. Imaging tests, such as a sonogram, also help your health care provider to reach a diagnosis.

Unlike fibroids that develop in other positions on or inside the uterus, submucosal fibroids tend to have a substantial number of blood vessels on their surfaces that can bleed. They also tend to prevent the uterine muscle's ability to properly contract because they distort the shape and function of the organ. Another noteworthy feature of submucosal fibroid tumors is their ability to grow to a size that obstructs the fallopian tubes, thus preventing passage of an egg in its journey to the uterus. But the story doesn't end there. These fibroids distort the uterine lining as they grow, causing menstrual irregularities. They may even become pedunculated and project into the cervix or even the vagina. As the growth moves about, because it is on a stalk and can twist and turn, it becomes a source of pain as well as abnormal bleeding. It is common for doctors to diagnose and remove submucosal fibroids that are the size of tennis balls.

Submucosal fibroids present many dilemmas for women and their doctors. They can be removed individually in a surgery called a **myomectomy**, or the fibroid and the uterus can be removed together in a hysterectomy. Hysterectomies have been recommended when women have multiple submucosal fibroids and excessive uterine bleeding.

biopsy

A surgical procedure in which a tiny sample of tissue is removed so that the cells can be viewed under a microscope and analyzed.

myomectomy

A type of surgery to remove an individual fibroid.

33. Why do fibroids cause infertility and miscarriages? When pregnancy does occur, what happens to the fibroid?

For most women, fibroids do *not* cause problems with fertility or pregnancy. However, when the growths do become troublesome, they can interfere with conception and progression of the pregnancy. In both of those instances, fibroids can become a source of emotional pain, especially when there have been multiple attempts to conceive. In addition to their capacity to prevent conception or lead to miscarriages in some cases, fibroids also can interfere with the birth of a baby when a pregnancy is otherwise successful.

To better understand how fibroids can become so problematic, it is important to know a bit more about their structure and function. Fibroids can make it difficult to get pregnant because, quite simply, they may act as obstructions that interfere with the normal processes of conception. There is no single way in which they do this. As mentioned in Question #32, submucosal fibroids can distort the shape and function of the uterus. A fibroid's potential to obstruct does not end there, however. A fibroid can interfere with the progress of a pregnancy by taking up the space needed for the fetus to grow. Finally, in instances when the pregnancy does proceed, fibroid growths can get in the way and hinder delivery of the baby.

These concepts are detailed below to further explain why fibroids make conception, pregnancy, and delivery difficult.

As a result of changing the shape of the uterus, a fibroid (or fibroids) can impede the sperm's path in the uterus as it travels to reach an awaiting egg. To picture this a little better, think of the vagina, cervix, and uterus as being in alignment with one another. When fibroids develop in between uterine walls, on the outside of the organ, or even within its cavity, its shape can become distorted, making the uterus no longer in alignment with the other structures. The growths therefore serve as roadblocks as sperm cells attempt to travel upstream to meet an egg. Large fibroids can block the fallopian tubes, interfering with an egg's movement toward the uterus. There are still other reasons why fibroids can interfere with conception and pregnancy: growths that develop underneath the uterine lining can so distort the normal shape of the organ that it is difficult for an egg to implant. Even when a fertilized egg does manage to implant, it may not be able to remain until term because as the fibroid (or fibroids) continue to grow, they stretch and further change the shape of the uterus.

Fibroids grow larger during pregnancy but they do not multiply during pregnancy even in the face of higher estrogen production during that time. This has led some, but certainly not all, doctors to speculate that perhaps it is not higher levels of estrogen but pregnancy's greater blood supply that causes fibroids to grow during pregnancy. Fibroids are highly dependent on a copious blood supply even when women are not pregnant. So, when fibroids increase in size during pregnancy, either miscarriage or premature labor can occur. Should a pregnancy manage to reach full term, a problematic fibroid may prove so obstructive that its presence may necessitate a Caesarean birth. The reasons for this are numerous, and one resides in a fibroid's ability to interfere with uterine contractions. Another possibility is the potential for a fibroid to become so large that it blocks the birth canal, making it impossible for the baby to assume the proper position for delivery.

If you have had many miscarriages, your physician will probably want to determine whether fibroid tumors are a cause. It is important to note that while you may have fibroids, there are numerous reasons for infertility. You will want to undergo a thorough medical examination to determine exactly what is hampering your ability to conceive and carry a pregnancy to term. The difficulty may or may not be related to fibroid tumors.

34. What kinds of tests will my gynecologist perform to confirm the presence of fibroids?

There are several tests your gynecologist may order to confirm a diagnosis of fibroids. As with any medical condition, your physician will begin by taking a detailed medical history. During this time, you will be asked a number of questions about your general health; previous pregnancies (if any); your menstrual history; your experience with abnormal bleeding, pain, or other reproductive system issues; diet; previous illnesses; and other health-related conditions that run in your family, etc. Your gynecologist also will conduct a full pelvic examination that will provide a relatively strong sense of where in the uterus the growths are located.

As part of your diagnostic work-up, the doctor will include both a bimanual examination and a rectovaginal examination. Neither of these procedures should be strange to you because they are the exams your doctor normally conducts during your annual gynecological visit. In the **bimanual examination**, your physician places two lubricated gloved fingers into the vagina and pushes upward while at the same time, on the outside of the lower abdomen pressing down with the other hand. This action allows your gynecologist to feel any growths in the uterus or on the ovaries. In the **rectovaginal examination**, your doctor simultaneously places one lubricated gloved finger in the vagina and another in the rectum. This is an important test for pelvic abnormalities and ovarian cancer.

Along with a physical examination, your physician will want to inspect the uterus without making an incision. This is done through hysteroscopy, using a slender, lighted tube-like instrument with a tiny camera attachment. The hysteroscope is inserted through the vagina and the interior of your uterus can be seen on a monitor. Another choice is a laparoscopic inspection of the uterus. This is performed with a different type of slender instrument that is inserted through the vagina. As with hysteroscopy, your doctor can see where the fibroids are located and get a very good view of their size and the surrounding tissue. Both hysteroscopy and laparoscopy can be used therapeutically when fibroids are removed.

bimanual examination

A type of investigation used for diagnosis, where the physician places two lubricated gloved fingers into the vagina and pushes upward while at the same time, on the outside of the lower abdomen, presses down with the other hand; this action allows your gynecologist to feel any growths in the uterus or on the ovaries.

rectovaginal examination

A type of investigation used for diagnosis, where the physician simultaneously places one lubricated gloved finger in the vagina and another in the rectum; important test for pelvic abnormalities.

35. At what age do fibroids usually develop? Are they problematic throughout life?

Fibroids are diagnosed at any time between the ages of 25 and 45. The growths are not found in girls who have not begun to menstruate, which demonstrates in yet another way that fibroids are intricately linked to estrogen secretion. The growths rarely cause problems in post-menopausal women because lower levels of estrogen in circulation at that point in life are associated with fibroid shrinkage. Fibroid tumors pose concerns at various points throughout the reproductive years for a variety of reasons. As mentioned earlier, their tendency to cause abnormal uterine bleeding is a major concern during perimenopause because the tumors tend to soften and bleed due to declining levels of estrogen in circulation. A major concern at any age would be the sudden growth of fibroids. This would be particularly worrisome among women after menopause when the tumors should be markedly decreased in size. For younger women, the sudden increase in a fibroid's size may suggest pregnancy. For older women, the sudden growth could suggest the presence of a malignancy, an issue that should be investigated immediately.

36. Are there ethnic differences underlying who develops fibroids?

African-American women are two to three times more likely to develop fibroids than Caucasian women, according to epidemiological studies conducted by the Centers for Disease Control and Prevention (CDC). As a result of that difference, black women are also more likely than other groups of women in the United States to have a hysterectomy because of problematic fibroids, and to undergo the surgery at a slightly younger age, usually in their mid-30s. The reason for a greater fibroid prevalence among African Americans remains unknown.

Epidemiologists who have tried to tease out why black women are more likely to develop fibroids also have found that women in Africa are not very likely to develop the growths. It suggests that something unique may be occurring among African Americans. These differences in incidence naturally raise questions about the interactions of hormone secretion levels, environment, and genetics, and are the same puzzling factors that scientists have tried to link in attempts to provide a unified theory to explain the cause of fibroids in all women. The reason for a greater number of hysterectomies in black women raises still other questions: Are the growths uniformly more problematic in African Americans, or are black women more likely to seek or be offered hysterectomies before first trying alternate procedures? No studies have yet offered definitive answers to those questions.

37. Do women tend to develop only one fibroid or can they occur in multiples? Where do they grow in the uterus?

Fibroids usually occur as multiple tumors and are without question the most common uterine mass in women of reproductive age. Some women can have as many as 20 or more of the growths in or on the uterus, and these tumors may occur in a variety of sizes. Some may be large, others small, some pedunculated, and still others burrowed under the endometrium. But just because numerous growths have developed within or on the uterus, that does not mean all of them are problematic, or that you must seek treatment for them if they are not producing symptoms or interfering with your attempts to become pregnant. With that in mind, in instances when the growths are causing symptoms—especially heavy bleeding that has led to anemia—you still would be wise to start treatment with the least invasive procedure. When attempts to remove individual tumors or to shrink them with medication prove too difficult or virtually impossible, your gynecologist may recommend a hysterectomy, especially when abnormal bleeding leads to severe anemia.

As mentioned earlier, fibroids can grow anywhere inside the uterine cavity, on its surface, or between its walls. There are technical names for fibroids that grow in each of those sites, and there are often site-specific problems when it comes to fibroids. Earlier in the discussion we mentioned submucosal fibroids (which are also known as intracavity myomas and intracavity fibroids). These growths are often associated with cramping, excessive bleeding, miscarriages, and infertility. Fibroids that grow on the outer surface of the uterus are known as **subserosal fibroids** and are noteworthy because of their tendency to be pedunculated, to grow on a pedicle—a stalk—that can twist and turn with normal body movements. They are associated with pain, especially when they press against the bladder, bowel or other pelvic structures. A final type of fibroid is known as an **intramural fibroid**, which grows between the smooth muscular walls of the uterus and can cause symptoms similar to submucosal and subserosal fibroids. Other types of fibroids include an **interligamentous fibroid**, which is a type of growth that develops within a ligament that supports the uterus in the pelvic area; and, the rarest fibroid of all, a **parasitic fibroid**, a growth that develops outside of the uterus, such as on the pelvic wall.

subserosal fibroid

A type of fibroid that grows on the outer surface of the uterus and has a tendency to become pedunculated (or grow on a pedicle or stalk).

intramural fibroid

A type of fibroid that grows between the smooth muscular walls of the uterus; may cause symptoms similar to submucosal and subserosal fibroids.

interligamentous fibroid

A type of growth that develops within a ligament that supports the uterus in the pelvic area.

parasitic fibroid

A growth that develops outside of the uterus, such as on the pelvic wall.

83

38. Are fibroids troublesome only during reproductive years or do they continue to be problematic after menopause?

After menopause, fibroids (and the uterus itself) shrink, ending for some women a tumultuous period in life during which they seemed to be in a pitched battle with their bodies. The fact that women do not suffer from problematic fibroids during the post-menopausal years strongly reinforces the notion that fibroids are highly dependent on cycling estrogens for sustenance and growth. For a majority of women, the end of their reproductive years offers a reprieve from fibroid tumors. Doctors are also aware that even the influence of estrogen in hormone replacement therapy (HRT) usually does not prompt the growth of fibroids in most women after menopause, which suggests the benign tumors may require a specific amount of estrogen in circulation to sustain themselves. Some women on HRT immediately after menopause may experience some growth of their fibroids. But again, the dose is so low in the pills that marked growth and a resumption of severe symptoms generally does not occur.

39. I eat plenty of green vegetables, do aerobics at the gym three times a week, and believe that I have a healthy lifestyle. Why do I have fibroids?

Unfortunately, there is no diet or exercise regimen that has been developed to prevent fibroids, although a small study from Italy suggests that women who include more green vegetables in their diets have fewer troublesome fibroids than do those whose diets are dominated by red meat. While that study has produced an intriguing hypothesis, no one has definitively answered whether certain dietary regimens can help women live their lives free of uterine fibroids. It also is important to emphasize that because fibroids are so pervasive and affect a wide range of women across a variety of dietary practices and cultures, it is clear that no single food or groups of foods have been found to prevent them or lessen their severity. That said, it is important to eat a balanced diet to ensure that you are receiving proper nutrients and minerals from foods, particularly if you are experiencing abnormal bleeding. It is vital to obtain sufficient iron to help combat the effects of anemia.

With respect to exercise, medical researchers have not found that a rigorous exercise program can prevent fibroid tumors. Intuitively, it would seem that rigorous exercise might help limit fibroid development and growth because exercise lowers estrogen levels (theoretically lowering the amount of estrogen that fibroids can use as fuel). But no one has yet developed an exercise regimen that is capable of limiting the ill effects of uterine fibroids.

This is not to discredit the value of exercise. Exercise can help you better cope with stress and especially the stress induced by a chronic medical condition, if you have fibroids that are causing abnormal uterine bleeding.

40. Does body weight determine whether you develop fibroids or avoid them?

Although there is some evidence that overweight women are more likely to develop fibroids than women who are thin, theoretically, because of potentially more estrogen in circulation, fibroids actually occur among many women of reproductive age, regardless of their body mass index (BMI). The growths are not limited to a single segment of the population. Fibroids are diagnosed across a spectrum of BMIs. Secretary of State Condoleezza Rice, who is a trim woman in her 50s, was treated for the growths. She is reported to adhere to a very rigorous exercise routine. Rice was relieved of chronic problems with fibroids in 2004 through an alternate procedure that allowed her to avoid a hysterectomy and to return to work within a matter of days. The procedure that Rice underwent is described in greater detail in Question #48.

When the growths are problematic, they cause abnormal bleeding and pain regardless of the number on a patient's bathroom scale. Nevertheless, scientists are searching for clues to find the variables that may prove to be risk factors for fibroids. Knowing these factors may one day help doctors predict which patients are most likely to develop the growths. The hope among scientists and physicians is that once risks can be identified, women at highest risk can take steps to avoid them. Even if excess body weight turns out to be a risk factor, there are likely to be many others as well, which reiterates the notion that more than one risk factor may underlie the development of uterine fibroids.

41. I have several uterine fibroids. Does that mean I need a hysterectomy?

No, it doesn't necessarily mean that hysterectomy is the right option for you. Hysterectomy is an appropriate option for some women with extremely problematic fibroid tumors, but certainly not all. As mentioned earlier, many women live with fibroids and never experience symptoms. A procedure known as myomectomy, which will be discussed in greater detail in Questions #43 and #47, is a form of surgery that allows your doctor to remove individual fibroids while preserving the uterus and the capability to become pregnant. However, when a uterus is riddled with many fibroids, it may be virtually impossible to remove each one individually and preserve the integrity of the uterus. In such an instance, especially when bleeding is prolonged and profuse, and other treatments have failed, a hysterectomy might be the best choice. Still, it cannot be repeated enough: Before resorting to invasive surgery, your doctor will likely offer more than one alternate procedure in an attempt to address your problem conservatively.

42. What are the main points I need to know about fibroid tumors? When would a hysterectomy be warranted because of them?

There are several key points that you need to know about fibroids. Some of these quick facts highlight many of the mysteries that remain to be solved about these growths.

A. *No one knows why fibroids form.* The tumors do not occur in young girls who have not reached puberty, and it is only after years of exposure to cycling estrogens that these knotty, fibrous growths appear.

B. *A majority of women experience no problems with fibroids.* Only about 25% of women have abnormal uterine bleeding, pain, or both as a result of the growths. Still others complain of no pain or bleeding but a protruding abdomen. Abnormal bleeding is the primary problem with fibroids that women report toward the end of their reproductive years. Researchers have no idea how many women actually have fibroids but some estimates are as high as 80% of all women of childbearing age.

C. *The tumors can cause infertility and miscarriages in some women.*

D. *Fibroids grow very rapidly during pregnancy.* During this time, a woman's blood supply increases and higher levels of estrogen are in circulation.

E. *The growths tend to diminish with menopause.* Scientists believe that this may be due to the dramatically lower levels of estrogen in circulation.

F. *Fibroids tend to grow in clusters.* Often there is more than one found in the uterus at the time of diagnosis.

None of the above factors on its own suggests that a hysterectomy is required or inevitable. You will also want to ask your health care provider about alternate treatments and which one or combination of therapies will best treat your condition.

43. What alternatives to hysterectomy exist for problematic fibroids? Is there a reliable first-step approach that doctors recommend before advancing to other treatments?

Therapeutic approaches to fibroids are highly individualized and depend on the symptoms you are experiencing, your age, whether you want to have children, and what you as a patient are comfortable with doing. Approaches recommended to women with uterine fibroids range from the simplistic to the high tech.

Watchful waiting is an important first step that your doctor is likely to recommend if you can cope with fibroids that may be producing symptoms, but the problems are not difficult for you to handle on your own. If you are not experiencing severe bleeding, if the pain is not unbearable, and if you are nearing menopause, it is likely that troublesome fibroids may resolve on their own as your ovarian activity declines. Watchful waiting is one way to avoid costly medical interventions and any side effects from potent medications.

If you are experiencing severe anemia, pain, and bowel or urinary incontinence, then you may want to consider any one or more of several approaches that are available to you.

For women who occasionally experience pelvic pain caused by uterine fibroids, over-the-counter pain relievers often help manage the discomfort. Your health care provider may prescribe something stronger for temporary pain relief when less potent medications do not seem to address the degree of pain.

Other options may involve more time to ponder on your part. Doctors can help alleviate some of the bleeding problems associated with fibroids by prescribing hormone-based medications. Certain **birth control medications** serve as a counterpoint to ovarian estrogen production. Another group of medications are known as **gonadotrophin-releasing hormone agonists (GnRHa)**. They prevent the body from making estrogen and progesterone. These medications can actually help reduce the size of fibroids by creating a pseudo-state of menopause. Another choice in this category is **mifepristone**, a hormone-based medication capable of slowing and sometimes stopping fibroid growth.

birth control medications

Hormone-based drugs used primarily to prevent conception. Also used as treatments for fibroids and other reproductive system disorders.

gonadotrophin-releasing hormone agonists (GnRHa)

A group of medications that prevent the body from making estrogen and progesterone. These medications can be prescribed to help to reduce the size of fibroid tumors by creating a pseudo-state of menopause.

mifepristone

A synthetic steroid hormone that blocks the action of progesterone; used in a few small studies of women with fibroids; capable of slowing or sometimes stopping fibroid growth.

Invasive alternatives to hysterectomy include myomectomy, which is a surgical procedure aimed at preserving fertility while removing the fibroids. A myomectomy can be performed with the aid of a hysteroscope, a rectoscope, or a laparoscope. The surgery also can be performed through an abdominal incision.

Uterine artery embolization is a technique that blocks the blood supply to problematic fibroids and is gaining favor among physicians and patients. Another innovative procedure is called magnetic resonance imaging (MRI)-guided ultrasound, which uses magnetic resonance imaging to pinpoint the fibroid's location and employs ultrasound waves to heat fibroids and destroy them. Two other surgical procedures may enter the discussion between you and your physician: **myolysis**, a procedure in which the blood supply to fibroids is halted, causing the fibroids to shrink and die; and **cryomyolysis**, a method of freezing fibroids, also forcing them to shrink.

uterine artery embolization

A surgical technique that blocks the blood supply to problematic fibroids.

myolysis

A surgical procedure in which the blood supply to fibroids is halted, causing fibroids to shrink and die.

cryomyolysis

A surgical method that involves freezing fibroids, which forces them to shrink.

44. What kinds of pain relief medications can be prescribed to cope with problem fibroids?

An appropriate medication can be chosen from a range of drug classes to treat the pain caused by uterine fibroids. Your doctor may recommend something easily recognizable to you that can be purchased at your local pharmacy or supermarket. Your health care provider may suggest acetaminophen (sold as Tylenol) for temporary relief from fibroid-induced pain or a nonsteroidal anti-inflammatory drug (NSAID), which is the class of drugs that include many medicine cabinet standbys: Motrin, Aleve, Naprosyn and, the original class member, aspirin.

If an over-the-counter medication does not address your level of discomfort, your health care provider can prescribe something stronger. Your doctor will need honest answers about the degree and frequency of pain you are experiencing to prescribe the medication that will best suit you.

Your doctor has many medications from which to choose, including prescription-grade acetaminophen and NSAIDs as well as medications from additional drug classes.

45. How can contraceptives help improve my problems with fibroids when it is already known that birth control medications can make fibroids grow?

Contraceptives may play a variety of therapeutic roles as they help to relieve certain reproductive system problems when the chemical composition of a medication is tipped in favor of a specific hormone. This is as true when treating uterine fibroids as it is when treating other disorders, especially endometriosis. Your doctor has a range of choices when it comes to the chemical composition of contraceptives aimed at controlling the bleeding spurred by rogue fibroids. Depo-Provera, a birth control medication composed of progesterone and given as an injection in your arm or buttocks is one way to approach fibroids, because the drug can help regulate the menstrual cycle. Your doctor also might choose the Intrauterine Device (IUD), Mirena, which consists of the hormone levonorgestrel. Neither of these options has an impact on the size of fibroid tumors. Only drugs that force the body into a pseudo-state of menopause can actually influence fibroids to shrink. Those medications,

Only drugs that force the body into a pseudo-state of menopause can actually influence fibroids to shrink.

which include the powerful class of medications called
GnRH agonists, are discussed in greater detail in Question #48. You may find it interesting to note that long
ago, contraceptives were not options for women with
uterine fibroids because of the medications' high estrogen content. The estrogen dose in the pills was so high
that it stimulated fibroid growth. As a result, some
women experienced rapid growth of their fibroids while
they were taking the pills, a situation that may have con-
tributed to an increase in the number of hysterectomies.

46. How do gonadotrophin-releasing hormone agonists (GnRHa) work? Is it similar to the action of mifepristone?

There are drugs that can be used in the treatment
of problematic fibroids that reduce the size of the
growths by homing in on the activity of hormones.
Gonadotropin-releasing hormone agonists (sold as
Zoladex, Synarel, and Lupron Depot) put the body in a
pseudo-menopausal state by reducing the concentration
of ovarian hormones (both estrogen and progesterone).
This forces the fibroids to shrink and lessens abnormal
bleeding, which in turn improves problems with anemia. This shrinkage is not always permanent. But some
gynecologists prescribe the medications as a first step to
reduce fibroid size. As a second step, they surgically
remove the growths.

One advantage to taking such medications is found in
their capacity to "fool" fibroids into sensing that
menopause has ensued, thus breaking the fibroids' pattern of growth. Instead of having a steady "diet" of
hormones, particularly estrogen, available as fuel, the
dramatically diminished amount of hormones in circu-

lation can force fibroids into retreat. In some cases, treatment with a GnRHa drug is all that is needed. The fibroids shrink and problems associated with them disappear. Such, however, is not always the case because fibroids can reappear, despite treatment with such potent medications. These drugs may cause a loss of mineral in the bones and subsequently are only prescribed for six months.

These drugs are not benign. They produce powerful side effects and cannot be used over long periods. The usual period of treatment runs about three to six months. Because the medications force women into a chemically induced state of menopause, they can trigger hot flashes, vaginal dryness, and mood swings. Some patients are unable to tolerate such side effects, and end treatment before the drugs have been used for a sufficient amount of time to have an effect. Certainly, though, this is not always the case because some patients have benefited from treatment, having experienced substantial shrinkage of their fibroids while preserving their uterus and reproductive capability. Going this route will require some discussion with your doctor about the risks and benefits. If you are interested in becoming pregnant and are planning surgery to remove shrunken fibroids, then you may have even more incentive to stay the course. Only you will be able to make that decision.

Mifepristone is nothing like the GnRH agonists. You may recognize mifepristone by its more common name of RU486, the so-called "abortion drug," or by its other moniker, the "morning after pill." The medication was developed in France as an abortifacient. But an evolving group of studies (all of them quite small) suggests mifepristone may be beneficial for women with fibroids who want to preserve their fertility. These studies have demonstrated that the drug has the capacity to force fibroids to shrink. The drug is highly controversial because of its link to abortion. But it offers an entirely different approach to treating fibroid tumors. Mifepristone is a synthetic steroid hormone that blocks the action of progesterone. A study by researchers at the University of Rochester (New York) found that after six months of mifepristone treatment, women experienced fibroid shrinkage and far fewer symptoms. The drug blocks uterine receptors for progesterone, which forces fibroids to shrink.

47. My gynecologist is recommending myomectomy. Will this alternative to hysterectomy permanently eliminate my fibroids?

Myomectomy is a surgical procedure in which fibroids are removed individually, and it can be performed in one of several ways. The least invasive are the vaginal procedures, which involve the use of specialized instruments: a hysteroscope, a resectoscope, or a laparoscope. Minimally invasive laparoscopic surgery, which involves a small keyhole incision, is another approach, as is an open abdominal operation, or laparotomy. The aim of a myomectomy is to remove individual fibroids as a way to preserve the uterus. Any of the surgeries can be tedious, depending on the number of fibroids that are present and where they are found in the uterus. You also may want to note that fibroids have been known to return in some women who have had myomectomies. If you are planning to undergo one of the vaginal procedures, you will probably want to seek out an endoscopic surgeon who has performed many of the procedures. About 40,000 myomectomies are performed annually in the United States compared with 200,000 hysterectomies for uterine fibroids. Many women who choose myomectomy do so because they hope to become pregnant. But the National Uterine Fibroid Foundation suggests the procedure also may be helpful for women nearing menopause who, because of a decline in cycling ovarian hormones, probably wouldn't experience a fibroid resurgence.

Hysteroscopic-assisted myomectomy involves the aid of a slender, lighted tube-like instrument. The device is inserted through the vagina, so no incision is made in this procedure. It can be performed in an outpatient surgery center. Miniature instruments are used as part of the operation to remove fibroids (and/or uterine polyps when they are present). If you are to undergo operative hysteroscopy, you probably will be very familiar with the instrument that your doctor uses because it is the same employed in diagnostic hysteroscopy. Hysteroscopic myomectomy can be used in the removal of submucosal fibroids.

Another type of myomectomy that can be performed without making an incision is with an instrument called a resectoscope. A resectoscope actually is a hysteroscope but one equipped with a wire capable of emitting high-frequency electrical energy to remove the growths, generally submucosal fibroids. The instrument is inserted through the vagina. As in a conventional hysteroscopic myomectomy, a resectoscopic procedure also can be used to eliminate uterine polyps. Like the conventional procedure, a resectoscopic myomectomy can be performed in an outpatient surgery center.

Laparoscopic-assisted vaginal myomectomy is yet another procedure, but it can involve a small incision, called a colpotomy, which is made in the vagina. Fibroids are cut out of the uterus by way of laparoscopic assistance and then are removed through the vagina. When an incision is made in the vagina, the uterus moves back allowing the physician to remove the growth. This procedure often is simply called LAVM.

Laparoscopic myomectomy involves a small incision in the abdomen near the navel. Through the instrument, your doctor can see the uterus and other pelvic organs. This procedure is best for fibroids that are growing on the outside of the uterus. Pedunculated fibroids, those that grow on a stalk, can be removed in a laparoscopic myomectomy, and so can subserosal fibroids. Slender instruments allow your physician to remove individual growths.

An abdominal myomectomy, or laparotomy, is the oldest of all of the procedures and the most invasive, but the one in which fibroids of any size and location can be removed. The procedure can prove difficult and complicated, depending on how it is performed.

48. I've heard that some women are being successfully treated for problematic fibroids with uterine artery embolization. What is that?

Questions #43 to #46 discussed the medications that may be effective in helping women cope with troublesome fibroids. But the effectiveness of the drugs for many women lasts only while the medications are being taken. In time, the growths can reappear. Because doctors are well aware of the spectrum of problems associated with the medications, which may include hot flashes, potential loss of bone mass, and in time, possible fibroid resurgence, your physician may suggest an alternative procedure that shuts down the fibroids' blood supply.

The technique capable of accomplishing such a feat is called uterine artery embolization (UAE), or uterine fibroid embolization (UFE). Regardless of which term is used, the procedure is the same. By significantly reducing the fibroids' blood supply, the intended result is shrinkage of the growths. A key benefit of the procedure outside of its potential to alleviate abnormal bleeding is that it leaves the uterus intact. If you have heard about UAE and think that it may be an option worth considering, you will first want to fully discuss the procedure with your health care provider to find out if you would be a good candidate. There are numerous reasons some women are not considered for the procedure.

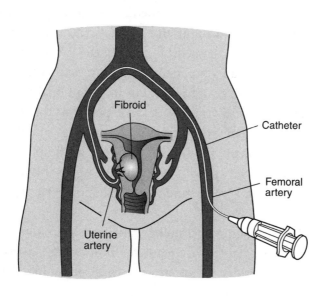

Uterine artery embolization usually is recommended in instances of excessive uterine bleeding and is widely recognized as an alternative to hysterectomy or myomectomy. Secretary of State Condoleezza Rice was treated for bothersome fibroids in 2004 through UAE. The technique is believed to be effective in 94% of patients, and is capable of relieving excessive bleeding and prompting fibroid shrinkage. Another advantage of UAE is that new fibroids do not develop. The procedure has been used to shrink fibroids of all sizes, including those that are the size of a grapefruit. While the technique has been used to treat fibroids of a wide range of sizes, doctors say UAE is most successful for growths that are under the size of a five-month pregnancy. The procedure affects all fibroids in the uterus, not just the one that may be causing abnormal bleeding.

Uterine artery embolization is minimally invasive and in some ways similar to heart catheterization because it not only involves guidance of a catheter through the femoral artery, it also must be performed with the aid of imaging technology. Before undergoing the procedure, your doctor will want a complete medical history, a pelvic examination, an ultrasound and magnetic resonance imaging (MRI). At most medical centers, the procedure is performed on an outpatient basis, but on occasion there may be an overnight stay. An interventional radiologist who is specially trained in UAE performs the technique in a hospital's department of radiology. Under local anesthesia, the physician's first step in the procedure is to make a very small incision in the upper thigh through which a catheter is guided to the femoral artery.

Using imaging technology, the physician can observe the movement of the catheter as it is guided from the femoral artery to the arteries that supply blood to the uterus. Releasing tiny particles that are as fine as grains of sand is the key to this procedure. The particles (called microspheres) are released into the uterine artery and the blockage they create is known as *embolization*. Just before the particles are released, an x-ray known as an arteriogram is taken. The arteriogram allows your physician to know precisely where the particles will lodge. The arteriogram essentially provides a roadmap for the microspheres' release. Once your doctor has read the roadmap, then he or she knows precisely where the particles are to be released. Tiny particles made of polyvinyl alcohol (PVA) are in actuality infinitesimal sponges. They are slowly injected into the uterine arteries. Small vessels feeding the fibroids tend to take up the particles first, causing these tributaries to be permanently blocked. The particles remain in the patient for life. Numerous studies indicate that the particles are "biocompatible," which means they are not rejected and do not cause irritation.

The uterine artery embolization technique has existed since 1975. At first it was largely performed in instances of obstetrical emergency, certain large pelvic malignancies, and pelvic fractures that produced excessive blood loss. With respect to fibroids, UAE was first tried in France to minimize abnormal bleeding in patients awaiting a myomectomy. Quite to the doctors' surprise, they noticed that for many patients, the fibroids shrank to an extent that completely eliminated the need for surgery. For most patients, this technique stops excessive abnormal uterine bleeding immediately. The fibroids themselves tend to shrink somewhat more gradually. Among the benefits associated with UAE is its shorter period of recovery, which is a few days compared with six weeks for hysterectomy.

The uterine artery embolization technique has existed since 1975.

Uterine artery embolization is not for everybody and though considered extremely safe, it is not free of side effects. The technique usually is not considered for women who plan to undergo treatment for infertility, nor is it recommended for women with chronic infections or those who have any contraindications to angiography. That technique involves making x-ray images of blood vessels after an injection of a radiopaque substance. Some people have allergic reactions to the contrast material used in angiography. Side effects may include nausea, fever, and cramping immediately after the procedure. Cramping may occur for a few days. Serious complications are rare but may include infections or uterine injury.

49. Please explain myolysis and cryomyolysis. These two alternates to hysterectomy sound very similar. How do they differ? Can they preserve fertility?

Unfortunately, neither of these treatments preserves fertility and they are not widely offered to patients. Both are geared toward eliminating troublesome fibroids that may be a source of excessive bleeding. While the two treatments are aimed at destroying uterine fibroids, they go about it in different ways. Both procedures are performed laparoscopically.

Myolysis is believed to work best on smaller fibroids and is not recommended for those that may have grown to the size of a cantaloupe. Treatment through myolysis allows your doctor to eliminate the fibroids' blood supply by using a laser or electrical current to cauterize (burn) the blood vessels feeding the growths. The technique usually is recommended to those who are not planning to have children because serious complications of pregnancy have been known to occur among women who have been treated with this technique. Theoretically, once the blood supply to the fibroid has been eliminated, the growth then shrivels and dies. However, there have been no long-term studies on myolysis.

Cryomyolysis is very similar except that it uses a supercooled probe to freeze the fibroids, which causes the growths to wither and die. A benefit is that it helps to prevent invasive surgery and removal of the uterus. Both procedures take about an hour to perform and patients do not have to be hospitalized. After either procedure, patients have reported abdominal pain and cramping. Their discomfort can be treated with mild painkillers. Recuperation requires a few days compared with six weeks for a hysterectomy.

50. I have heard my doctors use two terms, laparoscopy and laparotomy. What's the difference?

A laparoscope is an important device in the diagnosis and treatment of uterine fibroids and other reproductive system disorders. The instrument allows your surgeon to view your pelvic organs through a keyhole incision in the abdomen. The laparoscope also can aid surgery.

A laparotomy, on the other hand, is an open surgery involving an incision that is made through the abdominal wall. This is done either to conduct surgery, or to inspect the condition of the pelvic organs. In instances when fibroids are especially large or have grown in a complicated fashion, your doctor may recommend a laparotomy to help preserve the integrity of the uterus, if you are considering a myomectomy.

PART FIVE

Reproductive Disorders: Endometriosis and Pelvic Pain

51. What is endometriosis?

As mentioned earlier in this book, endometriosis is a condition in which uterine tissue becomes implanted outside of the uterus and deposits itself throughout the pelvic area, and even in more distant sites throughout the body. The disorder can cause inflammation, scarring, and a spectrum of other problems, the most notable of which is pain. Endometriosis affects an estimated 5 million women of childbearing age in the United States and is the second leading reason for hysterectomies, accounting for 19% of the operations that are performed annually.

Symptoms associated with endometriosis can run the gamut from mild to severe and may include diarrhea, painful bowel movements, and lower back pain during menstrual periods. But this complex condition also may prove problematic beyond the time of menstrual cycles, producing constant abdominal pain, pain during sexual intercourse, and underlying infertility. A majority of women are affected during their reproductive years, but some patients have been known to suffer with symptoms of endometriosis well into their postmenopausal lives.

Doctors usually diagnose endometriosis based on its stage. Mild endometriosis may produce few, if any, problems. Symptoms tend to escalate, though, with more involved forms of the condition, which may be designated as moderate to quite advanced. In the case of advanced endometriosis (or just "endo" as some patients more familiarly refer to it), excruciating pain, fatigue, and bloating may be the most persistent and dominant symptoms.

Regardless of the degree to which the disorder is affecting you, medical scientists know that the condition is driven by estrogen, which acts as a fuel influencing the activity of the endometrial implants and causes them to bleed. The disorder has proved mystifying to researchers who are trying to delineate its causes and develop more advanced ways of treating it. One risk factor suggests a hereditary association because endometriosis is known to run in families. The disorder also seems to have an association with immune system activity. But no one can say with any certainty what the causes of endometriosis might be. More than a dozen theories have been advanced over the years, and it is likely that many more theories will be proposed before medical scientists definitively settle on a cause or causes.

You may find it interesting to note the type of tissue that becomes displaced in endometriosis and deposited in sites where it should not be is the same as that which lines the inside of the uterus: endometrial tissue. These renegade deposits, which are sometimes called islets or islands, once they are fixed in a non-uterine site, are subject to hormone stimulation and bleeding just like the lining of the uterus itself. While the chief problem is usually pain, the condition also may be linked to abnormal bleeding, which is a primary symptom among those with fibroids and abnormal menstrual periods.

Other conditions with similar symptoms that must be ruled out before a diagnosis of endometriosis can be made include: 1) **cervical polyps**, which are tiny growths that protrude inside the uterus and are a source of abnormal bleeding; 2) reproductive system cancers, which in more advanced stages produce the kind of lower abdominal pain that is often considered one of

cervical polyps

Tiny growths that protrude inside the uterus and may be a source of abnormal bleeding.

the signature symptoms of endometriosis; and 3) uterine infections and pelvic inflammatory disease (PID), two infectious conditions. Your gynecologist will be able to differentiate among these diagnoses and determine the best treatment regimen for you. It is important that you work with your gynecologist to obtain a proper diagnosis.

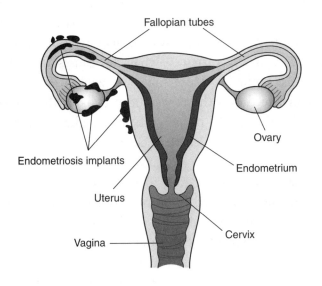

Displaced deposits, which are sometimes called "chocolate cysts" because of the way they appear upon close inspection through a laparoscope, can grow anywhere in the pelvic region. They can attach fallopian tubes, the outer side of the uterus or to the ovaries, leading, in some cases, to painful ovarian cysts. There are no physical differences between the endometrial tissue in the uterus and the endometrial tissue that may have implanted itself elsewhere. In addition to the ovaries and outer walls of the uterus, these renegade deposits may appear on the bladder, fallopian tubes, or sometimes as far north of the uterus as the lungs, but there is a difference in what happens when the tissue is stimulated monthly by estrogen. Endometrial tissue that lines the uterus has an escape hatch through the vagina each month when it is sloughed off as menstrual flow. When the renegade implants also bleed monthly on cue, there is no escape, so the blood then accumulates within the implants. These thickening islands of endometrial tissue can cause pain, inflammation, and scarring as they further imbed themselves into their adopted sites. If left untreated, the scarring may cause problems throughout the pelvic area, increasing for some women the intensity of what is often described as extraordinary pain.

For some women with endometriosis, there are no symptoms, a situation that leaves them unaware of the condition until they try to get pregnant. Only when the source of their infertility is discovered do they learn that endometrial implants have attached to the fallopian tubes and/or to the ovaries. For a great many women with the disorder, the implants cause **adhesions**, which are fibrous bands of tissue that abnormally cling to nearby structures. Adhesions cause major structures (perhaps an ovary, the outer wall of the uterus, or bladder) to become stuck together, a condition that can produce very dramatic pain.

52. What causes endometriosis?

The exact cause of endometriosis is unknown but there are some provocative theories that have been advanced. One notion suggests that **retrograde menstruation** may be a cause. Retrograde menstruation essentially is reverse menstruation. Instead of flowing out of the body, the blood backs up into the reproductive system, moving into the fallopian tubes and elsewhere throughout the pelvic region. So, instead of being discarded as menstrual waste, this extant residue from the uterus

adhesions

Fibrous bands of tissue that abnormally cling to nearby structures; may cause major structures (e.g., ovary, outer walls of the uterus and bladder) to become stuck together. The condition produces extraordinary pain.

retrograde menstruation

A theory that endometriosis is a process of reverse menstruation where, instead of flowing out of the body, the blood backs up into the reproductive system, moving into the fallopian tubes and elsewhere throughout the pelvic region. Instead of being discarded as menstrual waste, this residue from the uterus deposits itself throughout the pelvic area and continues to bleed and function as if it were still lining the uterus.

deposits itself helter-skelter throughout the pelvic area and continues to bleed and function as if it were still lining the uterus. Another theory, involving **vascular and/or lymphatic transport**, suggests that endometrial implants are carried to inappropriate sites in the body via the bloodstream, the lymphatic system, or both. This theory may explain why in some rare instances endometrial implants have been found in the small intestine, the lungs, and even more exceptionally rare, in the brain. Having a **hereditary predisposition** to the condition is another idea that has gained support. If your mother, sister, or other close relative has endometriosis, then it is more likely that you will be affected, too.

Some experts theorize that **immune system dysfunction** may explain why the disorder occurs, citing the failure of certain immune system cells to destroy leftover endometrial cells that are not ushered out of the body with menstrual flow. Yet another theory called **metaplasia** suggests that endometrial islands are deposited outside the uterus before birth, during the earliest phases of fetal development. As an adult, these deposits attempt to function as if they, too, are a uterus.

While theories abound, physicians and scientists underscore that no one knows for sure what causes endometriosis. No matter how the displaced implants arrive in their locations, they often can be found adhering to the bladder, the large intestine, and on major reproductive tract structures.

As discussed in Question #50, when endometrial deposits grow outside of the uterus, it irritates surrounding tissue, causing it to become inflamed and ultimately to develop scarlike bands of abnormal tissue known as adhesions. These can bind the pelvic organs together and result in excruciating cramps, heavy men-

vascular and/or lymphatic transport
A theory of endometriosis where endometrial implants are carried to inappropriate sites in the body via the bloodstream, the lymphatic system, or both.

If your mother, sister, or other close relative has endometriosis, then it is more likely that you will be affected, too.

hereditary predisposition
Suggests the likelihood that a medical condition has a familial link.

immune system dysfunction
A theory of endometriosis which suggests the disorder results from the immune system's failure to destroy any endometrial cells remaining after menstruation.

strual bleeding, and problems with both the bladder and bowel. Additional information on problems associated with endometriosis are discussed in Question #54.

53. At what age is endometriosis most likely diagnosed?

In some cases, endometriosis is diagnosed as early as the teen years, but the majority of cases are seen in women who are in their early 30s through their mid-40s. However, doctors now acknowledge that endometriosis is far more prevalent among teenagers than previously thought. Historically, it was believed that endometriosis was a disease of young career women who had postponed childbearing. We now know that nothing could be further from the truth, and medical science is beginning to produce more evidence about the disorder and the age groups it affects. The fact that endometriosis is seen in some post-menopausal women (though only a small fraction of those with the condition are past their reproductive years) only adds to the mystery. Virtually all other chronic reproductive system disorders end with the childbearing years, including fibroid tumors, which are far more pervasive and equally debilitating in some cases.

54. What are the symptoms of endometriosis?

Symptoms run a wide range. Some women may experience no symptoms whatsoever, even though there are deposits of endometrial tissue outside of the uterus. Others may have debilitating pain. The pain, of course, will depend on where the excess tissue has implanted itself and how extensively scar tissue has developed throughout the pelvic region. The list of symptoms, how-

metaplasia
A theory of endometriosis suggesting that endometrial islands are deposited outside of the uterus before birth, during the earliest phases of fetal development. As an adult, these deposits attempt to function as if they, too, are a uterus.

REPRODUCTIVE DISORDERS: ENDOMETRIOSIS AND PELVIC PAIN

ever, is long and some patients experience a combination of them. They include: backache, bloating, and pain when exercising, during intercourse, and bowel movements. Pain also may occur during urination, and urination may occur frequently because of pressure exerted on the bladder. Other symptoms include pain during and between menstrual periods and menstrual diarrhea.

As you can see, pain is one of the hallmark symptoms associated with endometriosis and it can be marked by excessive bleeding and bleeding at abnormal intervals. Legendary actress Marilyn Monroe is believed to have been severely affected by endometriosis. She was reported to have been so wracked with pain from the condition that on one occasion, while driving in her car, she pulled over to the side of the road, got out of the vehicle, and crouched by the roadside, incapacitated by the pain.

Perhaps more significant than the pain is the primary symptom of the disorder: infertility. Endometriosis is a leading cause of infertility and accounts for an estimated 30% to 40% of women who are unable to conceive. As mentioned in Questions #51 and #52, adhesions abnormally bind structures together and may also cause blockages in the fallopian tubes, making it impossible for eggs to pass. Of all the symptoms, infertility is the one that causes the most concern among patients with the condition.

55. How is endometriosis diagnosed?

As with any gynecologic condition, your physician will first want a full medical history, which will include detailed questions about your symptoms and the length of time you have experienced them. Bear in mind that many serious gynecologic conditions have similar symptoms. The pain and bleeding of endometriosis, when described, may seem to be no different than that caused by fibroids. So, your doctor will not be able to tell what you have until you have been thoroughly examined. Your further diagnostic workup will include a pelvic examination, which for some women with endometriosis can be painful. Your doctor very likely will want to perform a laparoscopy to view the extensiveness of the disease throughout the pelvic area. The disease is usually "staged" once your doctor has a sense of how limited or widespread it is in your body. The numbers 1 through 4 are assigned, with 4 signifying the most extensive disease.

56. I've been told that my endometriosis has produced scar tissue. Is this what is interfering with my fertility?

It is very likely that adhesions may be interfering with your fertility, but the only way to know for sure is to be fully examined by a gynecologist. Doctors know that endometriosis affects fertility in more ways than one. In addition to scarring that can occur, endometriosis also is known to decrease fertility by altering the chemical composition of fluid in fallopian tubes, which may cause the destruction of sperm. It is also possible that scarring has occurred within one or both tubes.

57. What alternate procedures are available for the treatment of endometriosis?

Doctors have a range of treatments from which to choose to address the problem of endometriosis. Treatments can be medications from any one of several drug classes; surgical treatments that preserve reproductive organs, or a combination of medications and surgical treatments. The simplest medication approach involves suppression of pain, as mentioned in Part 2 of this book. But your gynecologist also can choose medications that affect the balance of your two key hormones (estrogen and progesterone), or, if necessary, temporarily tamp down the flow of hormones, forcing you into a temporary state of menopause. Below is a list of a few of your physician's medication choices:

1. *Analgesics.* Controlling the pain is a primary concern among patients with problematic cases of endometriosis. Depending on the intensity of your discomfort, you may be able to relieve pain with such over-the-counter remedies as acetaminophen (Tylenol) or enteric-coated aspirin and other non-steroidal anti-inflammatory drugs (NSAIDs).

   Acetaminophen, while an analgesic, is not an NSAID and does not act directly on prostaglandins, the hormone-like compounds secreted by uterine and other tissues that are involved in pain and inflammation. Regardless of which over-the-counter remedy you choose, you must always carefully follow instructions on proper use that are included with the drug's packaging. Just because a drug is sold without a prescription does not mean that it can be taken with abandon. Non-prescription drugs come with caveats and side effects just like their prescription-grade counterparts. You should read the enclosed material to make yourself aware of any side effects.

With that said, you might find that over-the-counter medications work best for you, along with periodic check-ups from your health care provider. Keeping a handle on the problem in this manner may be all that you need. However, if your pain is far more intense and you find that over-the-counter medications are not strong enough, then your gynecologist may suggest turning to a more potent prescription medication. Many prescription-grade pain relievers are mentioned in Part 2. For extreme pain, and for a limited duration, your doctor may prescribe a narcotic pain reliever, such as codeine, oxycodone, morphine, or meperidine.

2. *Birth control pills.* Usually those with a high progestin (synthetic progesterone) content fit the bill best. Treatment generally runs about six months, but sometimes is slightly longer. Progesterone-based drugs trick the body into "thinking" a pregnancy has been established.

3. *Progesterone-only pills are another choice.* Oral forms include Provera, Megestrol, Avgestin, and Micronor. Your doctor also may recommend injections of Depo-Provera on a quarterly basis. All of these drugs act in a targeted fashion directly on the endometrial tissue, forcing it to shrink. Again, the theory behind the medications is tricking the body into the belief that pregnancy has occurred.

4. *Gonadotrophin-releasing hormone (GnRH) agonists* can be prescribed in a variety of ways: Lupron Depot, which is in this class, can be given as a monthly injection; Synarel is a nasal spray; and Zoladex is absorbed from an implant under the skin. These are the same drugs mentioned in Part 4 for

fibroids. They are prescribed for fibroids for the same basic reason that they are prescribed for endometriosis: they shut down a woman's hormone supply. With fibroids, these drugs stop the continued growth of these tumors. For those with endometriosis, GnRH agonists stop the further growth and damage caused by the disorder. As was mentioned in Part 4, GnRH agonists come with side effects. When your body is fooled into pseudo-menopause, it does not respond with just one or two menopausal symptoms; it is very likely that you will respond with the full battery. Your reaction to any of these drugs can be substantial: mood swings, vaginal dryness, hot flashes, night sweats, and short-term memory loss, so be prepared.

If your aim is to become pregnant, there are some recommendations that your doctor will probably make. Many tell their patients who are starting out on these medications not to attempt to get pregnant until the full course of the prescribed medication has been completed. The drugs usually are prescribed for a period of six to nine months. Most physicians suggest that patients attempt pregnancy about a couple of months after treatment stops and menstruation has resumed.

Even though these drugs induce a menopause-like state, and ovulation theoretically stops, there is still an outside chance that you might get pregnant while on them, so be careful. Your doctor very likely will advise that you or your partner use some form of birth control (condom, sponge, or other barrier method) while therapy is under way. Once your therapy is complete, you are free to resume sex without a contraceptive. Unfortunately, the cautions do not end there. Be aware that once treatment ends, endometriosis might come back. If that happens, you can begin another round of therapy.

58. What is danazol?

Danazol (Danacrine) is a synthetic male hormone capable of shutting down a woman's monthly cycle. Like the GnRH agonists discussed in Question #57, it creates a reversible state of menopause. Many women consider this drug to be frightening. It is very potent. Its side effects are also potent and can include changes in the timbre of your voice (it becomes deeper, not higher) as well as the commonly known side effects that are associated with menopause.

59. What are some of the surgical procedures short of hysterectomy that are aimed at helping women with endometriosis?

Laparoscopy has aided the diagnosis and treatment of many reproductive system disorders and endometriosis is no exception. The scope is inserted into the pelvic area through a keyhole-size incision that is no more than about an inch. Your doctor can then use it to see where throughout the pelvic area endometrial implants are deposited. Laparoscopy has become virtually indispensable. Various precision-driven instruments can be used along with a laparoscope to treat your condition. These methods include laparoscopic-aided laser surgery; laparoscopic-aided electrocautery (burning away unwanted tissue), and laparoscopic-aided surgery in which implants and adhesions are cut away. Any of these procedures can prove highly effective because they are minimally invasive. Once your doctor has gotten a bird's eye view of the endometrial implants through the laparoscope, the choice then can be made to vaporize, cauterize, or cut away the growths.

Laparoscopy has become virtually indispensable.

When laparoscopic surgery is performed to eliminate endometrial implants, the procedure is conducted with the patient under anesthesia. Through the keyhole incision, carbon dioxide is infused into the abdominal cavity to inflate it. This enlarges the space to permit an optimal view of the reproductive organs, the endometrial implants, and any adhesions that may have developed. The laparoscope itself is inside a thin, hollow tube, which is inserted through the incision. The scope's fiber-optic technology permits the abdominal interior to be viewed clearly on a monitor.

After inspecting your reproductive system, implants, and any adhesions, your doctor might want to eliminate the abnormalities with a laser. The device can be inserted through the same tube as the scope, or a second keyhole incision can be made and the laser inserted through it. A **laser** is a high-energy light source that emits a beam in a specified wavelength. It is capable of quickly vaporizing abnormalities with its heat. This high-tech, minimally invasive procedure not only allows for a same-day (or next-day) discharge from the hospital, it also allows for a smoother recovery when compared with more invasive surgical techniques.

By comparison, another procedure called a laparotomy will have a longer recovery period and is far more invasive because it involves opening the abdominal cavity. Your doctor may decide to perform a laparotomy if your test results reveal evidence of widespread endometrial implants and other abnormalities that often accompany endometriosis. For example, there may be numerous adhesions or the presence of ovarian cysts, which can create a far more complex disease state requiring a more invasive surgery.

laser

A high-energy light source that emits a beam in a specified wavelength. A laser can quickly vaporize abnormalities with its heat.

There are a few things you should know before under-going a laparotomy. As with any invasive procedure, there is likely to be significantly more pain than you would experience with laparoscopic surgery. In addition, the recovery period is longer, and the risk for infection higher because of the incision required to open up the abdominal cavity. Those cautions aside, the vast majority of women who undergo a laparotomy for endometriosis fare quite well afterward.

Finally, medication therapy and surgical treatment can be combined to enhance the likelihood that endome-trial implants can be eliminated, pain thwarted, menstrual cycles regulated, and fertility restored.

There also is an order in which doctors tend to recommend the two forms of treatment. You may first be given treatment with medication (a hormone-based drug) for about six weeks to attempt to shrink the implants. Once that is complete, your doctor then may proceed with a surgical procedure to remove as much endometrial tissue as possible. This may be followed with a prescription for birth control pills whose chemical balance is tilted toward progestin. Again, when these pills are prescribed to someone with endometriosis, the idea is to trick the body into reacting as if pregnancy has occurred. Treatment following such an approach can help keep endometriosis under control and further shrink any remaining islands of active disease.

60. How successful are alternative treatments? Can my fertility be restored?

Medical and surgical treatment can suppress endometrial growth and relieve pain for many women who are affected with mild-to-moderate endometriosis. Surgical removal of the implants and their attendant adhesions also can be very helpful, studies have demonstrated. However, medication therapy for severe endometriosis probably does little to boost the fertility rate.

Doctors do know that the milder the case, the more likely it is that pregnancy can be achieved. Severe endometriosis, on the other hand, can be exceptionally tenacious and a source of great anguish as women progress from one treatment to another, usually seeking both pain relief and restoration of fertility. As heartbreaking as the quest for relief has been for some patients, you should not assume doctors have given up on creative solutions to the enduring puzzles posed by endometriosis. For some women who have sought to restore fertility, artificial insemination has proved successful, but certainly not in a majority of cases. Experts have found insemination is most likely to be successful when pelvic organs have not become too scarred.

Other equally creative solutions are being tested in clinical trials involving a cross-section of patients. One potential treatment emerging from the domain of clinical research involves the breast cancer drug Femara (letrozole), which belongs to the class of medications known as aromatase inhibitors. When prescribed to women who have had breast cancer, the drug is aimed at keeping the disease from coming back. Femara may have a new role in the treatment of endometriosis by forcing the disease into retreat. It is being tested in combination with progestin, the synthetic form of progesterone, to provide a way of zeroing in on a key chemical reaction within endometrial implants.

An aromatase inhibitor is a type of drug that prevents the conversion of testosterone into estrogen by blocking the activity of the enzyme aromatase. By turning to a medication used to treat breast cancer, medical scientists are not saying that endometriosis has a relationship to tumor development, but that endometriosis, a disorder that thrives on estrogen, shares a chemical reaction with a form of breast cancer that also is driven by the hormone. The enzyme, scientists have discovered, is present in a variety of tissues throughout the body.

Endometrial implants, as it turns out, happens to be one of the tissues where the enzyme is abundantly found. Because the implants maintain such a rich supply of the enzymes, they are able to manufacture their own estrogen, which helps support their growth, thus exacerbating the pain and agony of endometriosis. Another way of looking at it is that endometrial implants essentially sustain themselves not only through the estrogen that is produced by the ovaries, but also through their own tiny and bustling estrogen factories.

Researchers from Northwestern Memorial Hospital in Chicago found that Femara may play a unique role in the treatment of endometriosis by borrowing a successful treatment strategy that has helped stave off breast cancer in those who are post-menopausal. Aromatase plays a pivotal role in post-menopausal breast cancer because it catalyzes a reaction in fat and other tissues that produce estrogen in women who are no longer producing a copious supply of the hormone from their ovaries. Femara initially was developed to treat advanced breast cancer but now is used to treat post-menopausal women with early-stage disease.

In a preliminary study, doctors put ten women on Femara and progestin for six months to see how well their endometriosis would respond. The women were also given calcium and vitamin D supplements because a side effect of Femara is bone loss. The women were selected for the study on the basis of having failed previous medical and surgical treatments for endometriosis. All had difficult cases of the disorder. Researchers theorized that if the production of estrogen could be stopped within the implants themselves, the endometriosis could be treated.

The research team, led by Dr. Serdar Bulun, conducted laparoscopic examinations on each woman before and after the study to determine the extent of their endometriosis and to gather a sense of how well the treatment worked. Bulun and colleagues concluded that the Femara and progestin regimen provided dramatic relief for patients. None had any evidence of endometriosis at the end of the study. Pelvic pain was reduced in nine out of the ten test subjects. The team reported its findings in the February 2004 issue of the medical journal Fertility and Sterility. The researchers have called for a larger study of this approach, which they believe may become first-line therapy for women with recalcitrant endometriosis.

61. Does endometriosis cause cancer?

Endometriosis does not cause cancer.

Endometriosis does not *cause* cancer. It does cause severe pain and infertility. Because so much about endometriosis remains a mystery, it has become a disorder that attracts scaremongers and fact-twisters. Of all the forms of cancer that one might expect to be related to the condition of endometrial cancer, researchers have found little relationship between the two diseases. Studies have shown that women with endometriosis have less than a 1% chance of developing the malignancy. Equally low levels of risk have been reported in most studies for cervical cancer. There have been mixed results from research involving ovarian cancer. Some studies determined that there was a very low risk and other results have shown a somewhat elevated risk. None of the investigations were large or rigorous, so it is perhaps best not to put too much credence into preliminary and inconclusive evidence. In addition, it is important to keep in mind that risk is all about chance and not destiny, a difference that often is misconstrued when the subject turns to cancer. There is an exceptionally rare malignancy called endometrioid cancer that has been seen in a few women who had been treated at some point in their lives for endometriosis, but even that disorder has a frequency among women with endometriosis of less than 1%.

62. Is there something that I can do to lessen the impact of endometriosis? Will exercise and changes in my diet help?

Unfortunately, there is not much that you can do outside of working closely with your gynecologist to effectively treat your condition. Exercising and maintaining a healthy diet may help lessen the severity of your symptoms, but doing these things will not "cure" endometriosis. Neither diet nor exercise effectively acts on the underlying nature of the disorder. With respect to diet, there are no foods that will make endometriosis go away. Some women have supplemented their diets with fish oil capsules based on the theory that fish oil acts weakly against prostaglandin activity. Prostaglandins, as stated elsewhere in this book, are the hormone-like compounds that are involved in pain and inflammation, the two key factors at the core of endometriosis. Again, you will want to discuss with your doctor what the addition of the capsules would mean in your case.

Your physician may say, "They can't hurt and they might help." But if your expectations are high and the capsules don't work (and that is a likely possibility), then you will have invested hope, time, and money in a treatment that, in the end, did nothing more than raise your level of anxiety. On the other hand, if you gain a reprieve from your symptoms, no matter how small or brief, then you are ahead of the game. Maintaining sound eating habits, in the meantime, is vital to overall good health.

Theoretically, exercise should provide some help in regulating your menstrual cycle, depending how often and how vigorously you exercise. Routine aerobic exercise is a major component of a healthy lifestyle, even for people who do not have endometriosis. But, again, don't expect miracles. Endometriosis is an exceptionally complex condition. Just as no single biologic activity is probably involved in its origin, no single action taken against it will suddenly make it vanish. So, you may want to think of tactics you take toward fine-tuning your dietary regimen and exercise routine as methods of better managing a chronic condition.

63. Is pregnancy possible after alternate treatments?

Many women treated for endometriosis are able to have children. In fact, the aim of alternate procedures is to eliminate problematic endometrial implants while preserving fertility, and leading patients to the day when they can have a take-home baby. Although doctors strive for that goal in as many patients as possible, unfortunately pregnancies cannot be achieved in all women treated for endometriosis. Endometriosis can cause extraordinary bouts of pain. Eliminating discomfort, in some instances, can be a primary focus of treatment. Some treatments, such as electrocautery, damage the uterine lining, which is needed to carry a pregnancy to term, making pregnancy after treatment impossible.

64. Does pregnancy "cure" endometriosis?

For generations, mothers of daughters with endometriosis have told their offspring about the curative powers of pregnancy. But the question about pregnancy and endometriosis is one with answers that have taken on lives of their own. The basic answer is, no, pregnancy does not cure endometriosis, but there are caveats and qualifiers. Women who have endometriosis can get pregnant but the endometriosis can return after the birth of the child. So you are not exactly cured of endometriosis if it has the capacity to return. Still, many women have declared themselves cured after they have given birth and found they no longer had problems with endometriosis. During pregnancy, endometriosis tends to improve because of the increased presence of progesterone, which forces implants into retreat. You may recall from earlier in Part 5 that progesterone treatments are administered because they mimic pregnancy. Doctors have had a measurable degree of success treating their patients with drugs that fool the body into sensing that a baby is on the way. To answer the question in yet another way, there is a kernel of truth to the notion of a "pregnancy cure." But the reality is more sobering. The disease not only can come back, it can do so and still trigger pain.

PART SIX

Additional Pain Syndromes

I have experienced excruciating abdominal pain.
My doctor has diagnosed adenomyosis.
Will I have to undergo a hysterectomy?

What is pelvic congestion syndrome?

More . . .

65. I have experienced excruciating abdominal pain. My doctor has diagnosed adenomyosis. Will I have to undergo a hysterectomy?

Not necessarily. There was a time when hysterectomies were routinely performed for adenomyosis and the diagnosis was confirmed only after the surgery had occurred. Now, with better methods of evaluating patients, alternate treatments are possible for many patients diagnosed with this relatively common condition. Still, it must be emphasized that hysterectomy remains an important treatment option because it stops what some women describe as excruciating pain.

adenomyosis

A very painful condition characterized by the infiltration of glandular tissue from the lining of the uterus into the muscular portion of the uterine walls.

Adenomyosis is characterized by the infiltration of glandular tissue from the lining of the uterus into the muscular portion of the uterine walls. Although the name adenomyosis may seem like another term for endometriosis because endometriosis is a disorder of displaced endometrial tissue, adenomyosis is a different condition altogether, even though one of its technical names is *endometriosis interna*.

Using today's more advanced techniques to view it, doctors say that the normal uterus tends to have a round, soft, beefy appearance. The infiltration of endometrial tissue into the muscle of the uterine walls forces the uterus to become engorged, causing it sometimes to double or even triple in size. While the appearance of the adenomyosis uterus can be quite dramatic, this relatively common condition causes symptoms in only a small percentage of patients. Some women are unaware of the condition until they are told they probably have it, following a routine pelvic examination.

Like endometriosis, the exact cause of adenomyosis is unknown, although there is evidence suggesting that women who have had children are more likely to develop adenomyosis than those who have not given birth. The precise percentage of women with adenomyosis also remains unknown. The disorder is typified by pain, which is the major symptom, but for some patients the disorder also may be associated with heavy menstrual bleeding, a tip off to your gynecologist that your problem is more likely to be adenomyosis than endometriosis. You may recall from Question #51 that endometrial tissue grows during your cycle and then is shed at the time of your monthly period. But in adenomyosis, the old tissue and blood is not efficiently sloughed off.

Among those who experience symptoms, cramping tends to occur along with heavy bleeding. Other symptoms may include spotting between periods, dull pain throughout the pelvic area, and a feeling of pressure on the bladder and rectum. Sexual intercourse can prove painful for some women. Adenomyosis is most often seen between the ages of 35 and 50. After your pelvic examination, a diagnosis of adenomyosis usually is confirmed through magnetic resonance imaging (MRI). On occasion, adenomyosis may be associated with a fibroid tumor. Any one who has suffered with a problematic fibroid knows the difficulty such growths can cause. To have one in connection with adenomyosis may seem unbearable. In instances of abnormal bleeding, your doctor also may consider a biopsy. But this invasive test most likely would be considered only to rule out other causes of pain and abnormal bleeding.

Adenomyosis is most often seen between the ages of 35 and 50.

Usually, GnRH agonist medications, such as Zoladex, Synarel, or Lupron Depot, are the first choice when medications are prescribed for adenomyosis because of their capacity to induce a pseudo-menopausal state, during which abnormal bleeding and pain tend to stop. Unfortunately, these medications are of only limited success in women with more advanced cases of the disorder. For them, there can be a resumption of symptoms once medical therapy ceases. But there are additional choices, especially if your hope is to avoid hysterectomy. A progesterone intrauterine device (IUD) is an approach that can help improve abnormal bleeding. Some doctors have prescribed birth control pills for women with adenomyosis to help regulate the menstrual cycle.

Another alternate to hysterectomy is hysteroscopic endometrial ablation. As explained in Question #59, hysteroscopic endometrial ablation is an outpatient procedure that is performed without making an incision. Your doctor inserts the telescopic hysteroscope through the vagina and into the uterus. The aim of endometrial ablation is to eliminate the uterine lining responsible for your monthly periods and to stop abnormal bleeding. Because the hysteroscope has a camera, your doctor will be able to view the inside of the uterus on a television monitor.

The procedure itself can involve any one of several types of ablation techniques: cryoablation, which involves freezing the endometrium to eliminate abnormal bleeding; or either of two energy sources, electrocautery or laser ablation. Any of the devices used to perform the ablation are inserted through the hysteroscope. After the procedure, patients are prescribed acetaminophen, ibuprofen, or naproxen to relieve any pain. You probably will be advised to refrain from putting anything inside the vagina for at least two weeks after the procedure, which generally means no douching, tampons, or sexual intercourse.

While endometrial ablation remains a choice for the treatment of adenomyosis, it would not be an appropriate treatment if you want to have a child. The treatment, regardless of whether your gynecologist uses a laser, freezing, or electrocautery, destroys the endometrium, which is vitally needed to carry a pregnancy to term. Some doctors, however, feel that ablation is an effective choice for women who do not want to have a hysterectomy or for whom the surgery would pose more risks than benefits.

Another alternate to a hysterectomy is removing an area of the uterus affected by adenomyosis when the condition is not widespread. When this is the choice, the procedures are: a laparoscopic myometrial resection, where a keyhole surgical approach is used; or open myometrial resection, where tissue is removed through a larger incision.

Despite the growing range of choices to treat adenomyosis, you may find when your symptoms are severe, and cramping and abnormal bleeding are unbearable, that your gynecologist may recommend a hysterectomy, especially if you no longer desire to have children.

66. What is pelvic congestion syndrome?

Another form of pelvic pain can occur before or during your periods and result from problems involving veins that nourish the pelvic area. Occasionally these veins can widen causing blood to pool in them, leading to the development of varicose veins and a condition known as **pelvic congestion syndrome**. It is estimated that as many as 15% of women of childbearing age probably have varicose veins in the pelvic area, and while most have no symptoms, others experience debilitating pain as a result of them. Among those who report symptoms, painful sexual intercourse is the complaint that usually brings them to their health care providers' offices.

Research suggests that estrogen may play a substantial role in the disorder because the hormone appears to be involved with the veins' widening. Patients treated for the condition describe their pain as ranging from dull to sharp. Some patients often speak of more penetrating pains that are sharp, stabbing sensations that tend to worsen at the end of the day, especially after hours spent sitting at a desk. Your doctor may suspect pelvic congestion syndrome after an extensive examination does not produce evidence of other pain-causing disorders, such as endometriosis or adenomyosis. Ultrasound imaging and possibly even magnetic resonance imaging can help confirm your health care provider's suspicions of pelvic congestion syndrome, following a pelvic examination and medical history. Generally, hysterectomy can be avoided for this condition. The most common treatment for pelvic congestion syndrome is a prescription for a pain-relief medication, usually a nonsteroidal anti-inflammatory drug (NSAID).

PART SEVEN

Reproductive Disorders: Uterine Prolapse

What is uterine prolapse and what causes it?

At what age is uterine prolapse usually diagnosed?

Will I have problems with other pelvic organs "relaxing" after a hysterectomy?

More . . .

67. What is uterine prolapse and what causes it?

Uterine prolapse, sometimes also called pelvic relaxation, occurs when the ligaments that hold the uterus and/or bladder in place weaken and loosen. In some cases, the weakening is so severe that the uterus and/or the bladder protrude into the vagina. Such extreme loss of elasticity can be caused by a number of factors: a congenital defect that leads to a weakening of the ligaments; successive childbirths; aging; and perhaps even a combination of those factors. A major symptom of the condition is pelvic area pressure caused by the protrusion of the uterus into the vagina. Uterine prolapse accounts for 16% of all hysterectomies performed in the United States each year.

Uterine prolapse accounts for 16% of all hysterectomies performed in the United States each year.

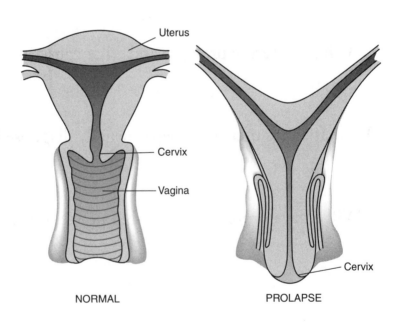

NORMAL   PROLAPSE

68. At what age is uterine prolapse usually diagnosed?

When it occurs, uterine prolapse is most often seen in post-menopausal women, although younger women who have many children in short succession as well as pre-menopausal women who are extremely obese also have been diagnosed with pelvic relaxation. The condition is noteworthy because of its significant impact on quality of life. Uterine prolapse is most often seen in patients who are older and overweight.

69. My doctor has told me to try a "pessary" as a temporary measure. What is that?

A **pessary** is a plastic device that, when placed in the vagina, helps support the uterus. Pessaries have been prescribed by doctors for decades to help women whose uterine ligaments can no longer hold the organ in its proper position. Such devices are not considered a permanent solution, however. When your doctor prescribes a pessary, it is viewed as a temporary measure because the device cannot change the lack of elasticity in your ligaments, which unfortunately can never resume their original taut condition. Most patients who are fitted for a pessary receive the device while under evaluation for a hysterectomy. In addition to uterine prolapse, pessaries also have been prescribed for urinary stress incontinence.

pessary
A plastic device that, when placed in the vagina, helps to support the uterus.

70. Will I have problems with other pelvic organs "relaxing" after a hysterectomy?

Generally, the answer is no because your only remaining pelvic organs after hysterectomy are the bladder and the vagina (and probably not the cervix because of the prolapse). As mentioned earlier, it is possible for ligaments that hold the bladder in place to lose tension and as a result it can fall. In fact, the reason that the bladder and uterus are sometimes diagnosed as both having protruded through the vagina in pelvic relaxation is because a bladder whose ligaments have loosened has put pressure on the uterus. Even though your bladder's ligaments may relax, this vital organ is not removed and actually can have more space in the pelvic region after a hysterectomy. You may find it interesting to note that the loss of elasticity in uterine prolapse does not happen overnight. The loss of ligament strength is gradual. Finally, if you had sagging abdominal muscles before your operation, that condition probably will not worsen as a result of hysterectomy, but could possibly improve if you follow a program of exercises focused on tightening that part of your body.

PART EIGHT

Reproductive Disorders: Pelvic Inflammatory Disease

What is pelvic inflammatory disease (PID)?
Is this condition dangerous?

What are some of the complications of PID
and how do doctors test for it?

What kinds of medications are used to treat PID?

More . . .

71. What is pelvic inflammatory disease? Is this condition dangerous?

Pelvic inflammatory disease (PID) is a chronic infection of the organs in the pelvic area. In its worst forms, PID not only produces physical scars in terms of the damage it causes but leaves many women emotionally devastated. More than 100,000 women a year become infertile in the United States because of chronic infections that have severely damaged reproductive structures. By definition, PID refers to an infection anywhere in the pelvic area, and although it is the persistence of an untreated chronic infection that most worries doctors, PID also can be an acute and temporary infection that can be effectively treated with antibiotics.

The National Institute of Allergy and Infectious Diseases, a division of the National Institutes of Health, estimates that 1 million women per year experience an episode of acute PID, with the rate highest among teenagers. Institute researchers estimate that about $7 billion is spent annually in the treatment of acute and chronic PID along with the numerous complications linked to the chronic form of the disease. Severe cases of PID have long been a reason for removal of individual structures of the reproductive system, such as one or both fallopian tubes or one or both ovaries. For decades, the infection also has been a major reason for hysterectomy, an operation that may be recommended when scarring and inflammation cause extensive damage throughout the pelvic area. Newer, less invasive techniques as well as the use of powerful antibiotics are helping some women avoid the surgery.

Any pelvic area structure, organ, or gland is vulnerable to PID. It can affect the fallopian tubes, uterus, ovaries, and in extreme cases can cause a narrowing of the cervix. A bout with PID usually begins as an acute sexually transmitted disease (STD) in which the disease-causing organism migrates upstream from the vagina to structures in the pelvic area. Most PID cases involve gonorrhea or chlamydia, two very common STDs. Gonorrhea, which is caused by the bacterium *Neisseria gonorrhoeae*, seems to have an affinity for the fallopian tubes, which is why in the not-too-distant past doctors largely thought of PID as primarily a disease of these two conduits. However, researchers have found that *Neisseria gonorrhoeae* tends to burrow into fallopian tube cells and then uses them as sites in which to multiply. As an infection mounts, delicate tissue in the fallopian tubes becomes inflamed and scarred. If the infection goes untreated, then the bacteria continue to spread, causing more inflammation and scarring as the process continues.

Chlamydia is a particularly worrisome infection because it can exist under-the-radar, so to speak, going undetected for years. There are many chlamydial subspecies, but the one associated with STDs is known scientifically as *Chlamydia trachomatis*. It is distressing that, while the infection is essentially silent for a relatively long period, as initially it produces few overt symptoms, the damage to reproductive organs ultimately can be quite extensive and results in a wide range of reproductive system complications. Public education campaigns about chlamydia have increased tremendously in recent years to alert people about the pathogen's dangers.

Regardless of the type of bacteria that causes it, when treatment is delayed and the infection advances, PID can result in inflammation, adhesions, scarring, pus-filled abscesses, and obstruction of the fallopian tubes. Adhesions (see Question #52) are abnormal bands of scar-like tissue that can cause nearby structures to unnaturally adhere to each other. Scar tissue is the damage left behind after extensive inflammation. Scar tissue can form on the inside and outside of structures, and especially inside the fallopian tubes where scarring can create blockages. When the tubes are blocked, eggs cannot make their journey to the uterus, so infertility results.

The National Institute of Allergy and Infectious Diseases also estimates that "a large proportion of the 70,000 ectopic (tubal) pregnancies that occur every year are due to the consequences of PID." One problem involving the disorder, especially with an insidious pathogen like chlamydia, the pelvic organs are vulnerable to secondary infections by other bacteria, which means some women develop one infection on top of another. Chronic PID, therefore, can involve multiple forms of bacteria that can become extraordinarily difficult to treat. In some situations patients must be admitted to a hospital and treated with medications intravenously. Indeed, resolving the infection over the long-term may prove an ongoing battle because extremely damaged tissues are readily vulnerable to re-infection.

Chronic cases are marked by adhesions that cause reproductive organs and other pelvic structures to adhere to each other by way of bands of scar-like tissue. The organs themselves can become encased in scar tissue and the bands of abnormal tissue can extend to include the bowel. With so much scarring, there are crevices in which pockets of pus and bacteria can lodge, remaining unscathed by antibiotics. These pathogens are capable of multiplying anew, spreading and causing intense infection again and again.

72. With such extensive scarring and inflammation associated with PID, what are the symptoms?

Symptoms of PID vary over a wide range depending on the degree of infection and the microbe causing the infection. They may include vaginal discharge, lower abdominal pain, and for some patients heavy menstrual bleeding and intermittent bleeding between periods. Additional symptoms are constipation because of the damage to the large intestine by adhesions. Fever is another sign of the disease, especially during acute phases when bacteria are particularly pervasive.

73. What are some of the complications of PID and how do doctors test for it?

One of the major complications, aside from those alluded to in Question #72, is the masses of pus called pelvic abscesses. Years ago these abscesses were treated surgically by removing a fallopian tube and its ovary. More recently, doctors have treated these complexes by draining them through a catheter or by eliminating them through keyhole laparoscopic surgery, which involves making a small incision in the abdomen to insert a device that is equipped with a tiny camera linked to a monitor; this allows the doctor to inspect pelvic organs without performing a more invasive operation (see Question #8).

Testing for PID is extensive and involves your doctor taking a detailed medical history. The reasons for this are in the best interests of your health. PID often occurs in combination with viral infections, such as HIV, hepatitis B and C, not to mention the secondary bacterial infections that can occur in instances when infection is extensive. Along with the medical history, your doctor will conduct a complete physical that includes a pelvic examination. Your gynecologist will also check for swollen lymph nodes, rashes, and other overt symptoms of infection. Laboratory tests will be extensive and will involve cultures taken from the pelvic area, blood tests, and urine analysis.

74. What kinds of medications are used to treat PID?

As mentioned in Question #71, antibiotics are the medications used for treatment of the bacterial species that have invaded pelvic structures. Antibiotics can be administered through an intravenous line should you be hospitalized for the condition. However, oral antibiotics are a more common form of treatment. Doctors generally choose what is often called a long-course of antibiotic treatment, which means your medication therapy can run six to eight weeks. In some instances, patients additionally may be prescribed a corticosteroid drug, usually prednisone. Corticosteroids are powerful anti-inflammatory agents and can be used to halt inflammatory processes in pelvic structures. Inflammation itself is mediated by the immune system, which causes the reddening and heat that flare in the midst of an attack by bacteria and other pathogens. Doctors also have found that the steroid drug helps the antibiotics reach small pockets of bacteria because, as inflammation subsides, there are fewer deep-seated sites for abscesses to form and bacteria to hide.

75. Is there any good news for women treated for PID?

The good news is that many patients with chronic PID can be treated without hysterectomy. Adhesions can be eliminated through precision microsurgical techniques. Removing adhesions is surgery that is extraordinarily tedious, but the bands of abnormal tissue can be eliminated, and even more surprising, if they are not too damaged the fallopian tubes can be repaired and even spared in some cases. However, it is important to underscore that such is the exception and not the rule. When infection has been extensive, attempts to save vital structures are not always possible. More often than not, years of chronic PID can cause a situation where neither tube is repairable. So while ultimately fertility is lost, the take-home message is that the infection was eliminated and your health restored.

Many patients with chronic PID can be treated without hysterectomy.

PART NINE

Reproductive Disorders: Pre-Cancerous and Cancerous Conditions of Reproductive Structures

Would a pre-cancerous condition be a reason
for a hysterectomy?

What about pre-cancerous conditions in the cervix?

What are the major forms of cancer that
can result in a hysterectomy?

More . . .

76. Would a pre-cancerous condition be a reason for a hysterectomy?

As the term implies, when magnified and studied under a microscope, pre-cancerous cells show changes that deviate from patterns of normal growth. It is likely that these conditions may never fully transform into cancer, but your health care provider undoubtedly will explain what the cell patterns mean and advise you whether closer monitoring of your case is warranted or whether a more aggressive approach—which may or may not mean a hysterectomy—is the best way to address your case.

Cancer is not a death sentence. Because of major scientific breakthroughs in imaging techniques and pharmaceuticals, many women are being cured of a variety of cancers. But it is crucial that the appropriate physical examination and tests are done to precisely identify the cells and their stage of development as soon as possible.

To further grasp some of the finer points regarding cellular growth conditions in the cervix and endometrium, it is best to step away from the world of medicine for a moment and review the structure of words. You may recall from Question #1 that the word *hyster*, the prefix to the word hysterectomy (meaning "womb"), has ancient roots. As it turns out, suffixes (the endings of words) are equally important because they reveal vital information about a word's meaning with respect to your health.

For example, the suffix *plasia* provides a lot of information regarding what a pathologist is viewing in tissue under a microscope. The suffix means "growth." Hyperplasia means overgrowth and dysplasia is disordered growth. Both words have important meanings regarding diagnoses of both endometrial and cervical tissues.

77. What is endometrial hyperplasia?

One term heard frequently is endometrial hyperplasia. It refers to an overgrowth of cells in the endometrium, which is the inner lining of the uterus. This proliferation of cells causes the endometrium to thicken. Not all diagnoses of endometrial hyperplasia are indicative of a pre-cancerous condition. Currently, about 5% of hysterectomies performed in the United States are done because of a diagnosis of pre-cancerous endometrial hyperplasia.

Understanding exactly what your diagnosis means will help put into perspective the various nuances that pathologists detect when viewing slides from any number of patients. Because one case of endometrial hyperplasia can differ significantly from the next, the treatment recommendation you receive may differ from that of a friend or close relative who also might have been diagnosed with the condition. One woman may receive a prescription for medication while another must undergo a hysterectomy because her diagnosis of endometrial hyperplasia suggests the presence of pre-cancerous cells. Your doctor will retrieve a tissue sample from you through any one of the following procedures: hysteroscopy and biopsy, or a dilation and curettage (D&C). The specimen will be sent to a pathologist to study and analyze.

Doctors have long known that endometrial hyperplasia occurs in the presence of continuous stimulation by estrogen. The stimulation, in turn, alters the usual balance between estrogen and progesterone, creating a chemical scenario that can have a profound impact on the inner lining of the uterus. There may be too much estrogen and too little progesterone. Women who have taken estrogen therapy alone without progestin as a treatment for menopausal symptoms have developed endometrial hyperplasia. The condition also may occur naturally much earlier in life in very young women whose menstrual cycles have not regulated. Their cycles are characterized by more estrogen than progesterone. Progesterone, you may recall from the questions in Part 3, is responsible for sloughing off the endometrial lining each month as menstrual flow. When there is not enough progesterone in circulation to perform that job, pain and abnormal bleeding can occur.

The overgrowth of cells that characterize endometrial hyperplasia can be either simple or complex. Endometrial tissue may be further characterized as exhibiting **atypia**, a term pathologists use to describe atypical (that is, abnormal) cells. A **simple hyperplasia** means there is an overgrowth of cells in the uterus. The inner lining of the uterus has become thick. Despite such cellular proliferation, the uterine structure remains unchanged and there is no evidence of atypical, pre-cancerous cells. Other terms used to describe simple hyperplasia are: mild, Swiss cheese, and cystic.

If your diagnosis is simple endometrial hyperplasia without atypia, rest assured there is no reason for alarm. Among diagnoses of the disorder, this one draws the lowest level of concern from gynecologists. Simple endometrial hyperplasia without atypia is not a pre-cancerous condition. This form of hyperplasia has been known, in some cases, to resolve on its own or

atypia

A term pathologists use to describe abnormal cells.

simple hyperplasia

A condition typified by an overgrowth of cells in the uterus; the inner lining of the uterus becomes thickened. Despite such cellular proliferation, the uterine structure remains unchanged and there is no evidence of atypical or pre-cancerous cells. Also called mild, Swiss cheese, and cystic.

REPRODUCTIVE DISORDERS: PRE-CANCEROUS AND CANCEROUS

following a D&C. So one course of action may be to perform a D&C. Additionally, your doctor may prescribe a progesterone-based medication, usually medroxyprogesterone acetate (Provera or Cycrin). Younger women may receive a prescription for birth control pills.

Another possible diagnosis is **simple endometrial hyperplasia with atypia**. Even though cells detected in the sample demonstrate an abnormality and possess about an 8% chance of becoming cancerous, the usual recommendation for patients is a D&C, progestin therapy, and periodic monitoring.

When the diagnosis is **complex hyperplasia**, again, there is an overgrowth of cells in the uterus, but with this condition the proliferation is so excessive that the structure of the uterus itself has changed. Under the microscope, the infinitesimal glands of the endometrium can be seen crowding one another and the endometrium's stroma cells also exhibit marked proliferation. The pathologist may have further described your case as adematous, glandular, or moderate hyperplasia, and adding yet a final note of *with* or *without* atypia.

The conclusion of *without atypia* means that the endometrium has thickened and the architecture of the endometrium has changed, but there is no evidence of pre-cancerous cells. When the diagnosis is complex hyperplasia without atypia, the usual course of action is a D&C along with a prescription of progesterone therapy for several months. Your doctor probably will want to take a tissue sampling from the endometrium at the end of your medication therapy to determine whether the condition has resolved and that no atypical cells are present.

simple endometrial hyperplasia with atypia

A term used by pathologists for cells that demonstrate an abnormality and possess about an 8% chance of becoming cancerous. The usual recommendation for patients is a D&C, progestin therapy, and periodic monitoring.

complex hyperplasia

A term used by pathologists to define an overgrowth of cells in the uterus where the proliferation is so excessive that the structure of the uterus itself has changed. Microscopically, the infinitesimal glands of the endometrium can be seen crowding one another. The endometrium's stroma cells also exhibit marked proliferation.

Patients who receive a diagnosis of complex hyperplasia with atypia have about a 25% to 30% chance of their cells progressing to endometrial cancer. This compares with a chance under 5% among those patients who receive a diagnosis of complex endometrial hyperplasia without atypia. Hysterectomy is strongly recommended for those with complex hyperplasia with atypia to lower the risk of the cells progressing further toward cancer. You might think of atypical cells this way: They are on the road to becoming cancerous, but have not yet reached that point. The purpose of a hysterectomy is to spare you the journey.

If you have received a diagnosis of endomentrial hyperplasia, you are encouraged to talk to your health care provider about the condition so that the various treatment methods can be made clear, and that you are aware of follow-up treatments and the need for any further monitoring.

cervical dysplasia

The abnormal growth of cells on the surface of the cervix (which is the entrance to the uterus).

cervical intraepithelial neoplasia (CIN)

A pre-cancerous condition caused by an abnormal growth of cells on the surface of the cervix. These cells can linger for long periods in a pre-cancerous state before advancing to invasive cancer.

78. What about pre-cancerous conditions in the cervix?

Cervical dysplasia refers to the abnormal growth of cells on the surface of the cervix, the entrance to the uterus. The pre-cancerous condition of concern in the cervix is known as **cervical intraepithelial neoplasia (CIN)**. Doctors have found that these cells can linger for long periods in a pre-cancerous state before advancing to invasive cancer. Pathologists look for a range of changes when classifying patients' specimens. Cervical cells can appear as: mild (CIN I); moderate to marked (CIN II); severe (CIN III); or they may be defined as carcinoma in situ (which is a localized cancer). CIN I to CIN III are pre-cancers.

As their numerical designations imply, each differs significantly. CIN I, for example, is likely to resolve on its own, and up to 70% of such cases do revert to a normal cell pattern. Such is not the case with all classifications. Even though pre-cancerous cells do not cause any symptoms, higher-grade dysplasias have the potential to progress toward cervical cancer in situ when left untreated. Ignoring their presence means that these cells will progress to become invasive cervical cancer. It can take up to a decade for the transformation to occur.

Treatment for CIN can involve any of the following: electrosurgical resection; a cone biopsy; or ablation of the abnormal tissue through laser treatment or cryotherapy. When CIN has progressed deeply into cervical tissue, your doctor may recommend a hysterectomy.

79. What are the major forms of cancer that can result in a hysterectomy?

Three major forms of cancer can affect the reproductive area: endometrial, cervical, and ovarian. Of the three, endometrial cancer is the most common reproductive malignancy, with more than 40,500 cases diagnosed annually in the United States, followed by ovarian cancer with 22,000 cases, and about 10,400 cases of cervical cancer. In underdeveloped regions of the world, cervical cancer stands out as a major health threat to women. Scientists are scrambling to perfect vaccines that promise to bring the global problem of cervical cancer under control. The disease is associated with infection by the sexually transmitted herpes papilloma virus, and because of high rates of cervical cancer throughout many countries, it is considered the most pervasive gynecologic cancer in the world.

Three major forms of cancer can affect the reproductive area: endometrial, cervical, and ovarian.

In the United States, gynecologic cancers, regardless where they occur in the pelvic region, account for about 10% of all hysterectomies. In addition to the most common sites of reproductive tract cancers, there are also rare malignancies that affect other structures and less common malignancies that cause pain. Cancer also can occur in the fallopian tubes (the conduits that propel eggs into the uterus), for example. A hysterectomy can be performed for any form of cancer that develops in the reproductive tract.

80. What facts should I know about endometrial cancer?

endometrial cancer

A malignancy that affects cells lining the uterus.

Endometrial cancer is a malignancy that affects the lining of the uterus. The incidence of this type of cancer rose in the United States between 1988 and 1998 before leveling off in 2001. In the United States, endometrial cancer is the fourth leading cause of cancer in women following breast, lung, and colorectal cancers. Most cases of endometrial cancer are diagnosed after menopause. As with all forms of cancer, a hysterectomy is an important procedure because it is performed to remove the malignancy from the body and to prevent the cancer from spreading elsewhere.

Abnormal bleeding and spotting are early signs of endometrial cancer and those symptoms often help your doctors detect the condition while it is in a treatable stage. We emphasized that if you have unusual bleeding or discharge, you should report the symptoms immediately to your health care provider. For younger women, abnormal bleeding and/or spotting may have any number of causes. But among post-menopausal women, abnormal bleeding may well be a signal of a gynecologic cancer. It is noteworthy that in a majority of cases, early symptoms involve abnormal bleeding, but for a small percentage of women there is a white vaginal discharge. Additional symptoms may include generalized pelvic pain, painful urination, and pain with intercourse. When earlier symptoms go unrecognized, pain usually is the first major sign that something has gone awry.

This type of cancer has been in the news in recent years with the cases of two high-profile women. Actress Fran Drescher was diagnosed with the cancer in 2000, and later embarked on a public awareness campaign, writing about her experiences in her book entitled *Cancer Schmancer*, and speaking out about early symptoms and ways of avoiding risks. Academy Award-winning actress Anne Bancroft died of the cancer in 2005 after a long battle with the disease.

Endometrial cancer is most likely caused by cumulative estrogen exposure, which in some cases may be related to estrogen replacement therapy, without the additional use of progestin (a synthetic version of progesterone), which protects the uterus. Additional risks include: use of the breast cancer drug tamoxifen; early menarche and late menopause; never giving birth; polycystic ovary syndrome; and obesity. The theory is that fat cells serve as production sites for estrogen among obese women, particularly those who are post-menopausal. With more estrogen in circulation, these women are believed at greater risk of cancer caused by additional years of exposure past menopause. Risk factors for endometrial cancer that are believed to be not quite as potent include infertility and hereditary non-polyposis colon cancer (HNPCC).

The good news about endometrial cancer is that it tends to be slow growing and often remains confined to the uterus. Stage 1 disease is successfully treated in the vast majority of patients. However, the disease can become more problematic if it spreads beyond the uterus. An estimated 7,300 women in the United States die annually as a result of advanced stage disease. Radiation therapy and drug treatment may be included as part of the overall treatment plan for the cancer. In addition to endometrial cancer (malignancy of the uterine lining), there is a rare form of uterine cancer that affects the smooth muscle of the uterine walls. This form of uterine cancer is known as a sarcoma and it has a reputation for rapid growth. This fast-moving cancer is capable of invading the endometrium. Sarcoma accounts for an estimated 2% to 4% of all cancers in the uterus.

81. I have cervical cancer and would like to have more children. Can just the cervix be removed?

This is a difficult question to answer because the treatment your doctor chooses is based on the findings of your tests, which define the extent of your cancer. In some instances, surgery may be local. That is, your doctor may remove only the abnormal tissue that is found within or near the cervix. If the disease has invaded deeper within the cervix but has not spread into the uterus, your doctor may choose to remove the tumor and surrounding tissue but leave the uterus and ovaries intact. But these are hypothetical situations based on the numerous ways in which cervical cancer occurs and how extensively the disease can develop. A woman may require a hysterectomy or she may even request a hysterectomy to provide the greatest assurance that the most extensive operation has been performed to guard against a recurrence of the cancer. When a hysterectomy is performed, the doctor removes the uterus, including the cervix, and probably the ovaries and fallopian tubes. Surrounding lymph nodes will also be removed.

82. What are the symptoms of ovarian cancer?

Ovarian cancer can be very subtle initially and often remains unnoticed until the disease has advanced, owing to the relatively vague and silent symptoms that may have been smoldering for months, if not years. Abdominal bloating is one symptom of the disease and flatulence is another. Both of those symptoms can be overlooked as any one of several conditions that most women would consider minor, such as menstrual issues, if you're still in your childbearing years, or gastrointestinal problems, no matter what your age. Spotting or heavier bleeding is the symptom that often causes women to seek a doctor's opinion. When the disease is discovered at an advanced stage, your doctors undoubtedly will advise you that the likelihood of conservative treatment measures are slim. The obvious surgical strategy against ovarian cancer is to eliminate the cancer. This can mean an extensive surgery because of the potentially life-threatening nature of the disease. All other considerations, unfortunately, are secondary.

83. I am still of childbearing age and have been diagnosed with ovarian cancer. Is there a fertility-sparing alternative for me?

A fertility-sparing surgery could be performed depending on the stage of your disease. Ovarian cancer often is treated aggressively because it is most likely to be found in an advanced stage. However, if you have been diagnosed with ovarian cancer, have not reached menopause, and are still entertaining the idea of having children, you should have a frank discussion with your physician about fertility-sparing surgery. If one ovary remains cancer-free you can consider freezing your eggs. This option has been offered to some women.

Such an operation would give you the option to have children in the future but allow your cancer to be treated immediately. This approach could involve removing only the affected ovary and its associated fallopian tube. It's important to bear in mind that such limited surgery is rare for ovarian cancer. The standard operation for ovarian cancer is **total abdominal hysterectomy with bilateral salpingo-oophorectomy (TAH-BSO)**, which is removal of the uterus, the fallopian tubes, and both ovaries, even though the cancer may have been detected in just one ovary. However, you may be a candidate for fertility-sparing surgery if your cancer has been detected in an early stage (usually stage 1 in a classification sys-

total abdominal hysterectomy with bilateral salpingo-oophorectomy (TAH-BSO)

A type of hysterectomy that involves the removal of the uterus, the fallopian tubes, and both ovaries.

tem that runs from stages 1 to 4), your cancer is not of an aggressive cell type, there is no evidence of the cancer in your lymph nodes, and there are no signs of cancer in the opposite ovary. Often it is difficult to give a clear-cut answer to patients immediately. For example, after a fertility-sparing operation is performed and if further pathologic study of the tumor reveals that it has characteristics of a more aggressive type of cancer, your doctor probably will recommend the TAH-BSO.

84. Does a hysterectomy cure ovarian cancer?

A hysterectomy is only one part of an extensive treatment regimen for ovarian cancer, and because it is a single treatment among several that are performed for the disease, hysterectomy alone is never seen as curative. Ovarian cancer is a very complex and unpredictable disease. Among cancers it is an extraordinarily difficult one to treat because it usually is diagnosed at a late stage, due to the vague symptoms produced early in its course. Hysterectomy is performed to eliminate all visible traces of the disease and to ensure that indolent cells are not left behind in other structures. A hysterectomy is only one in a series of treatments your **gynecologic oncologist** (a physician specializing in the types of cancer affecting the female reproductive structures) will likely recommend.

Ovarian cancer is a very complex and unpredictable disease.

gynecologic oncologist

A degreed (MD), board certified specialist trained in the physical, chemical, and biologic properties and features of neoplasms (cancers), including causation, pathogenesis, and treatment. Also trained as a gynecologist.

155

Getting a Diagnosis and a Second Opinion

Who are the appropriate health care providers for gynecologic conditions?

My insurance company says I need a second opinion. Will my gynecologist feel insulted?

How do I get a second opinion?

More . . .

85. Who are the appropriate health care providers for gynecologic conditions?

gynecologist

A degreed (MD), board certified specialist in disorders of the female reproductive tract as well as issues involving endocrinology and reproductive physiology.

A **gynecologist** is the specialist diagnosing and treating most of the conditions involving the female reproductive system. An **interventional radiologist** would be the physician providing treatments such as uterine artery embolization. If you are to have endoscopic surgery, you probably will want to see a gynecologist who specializes in those procedures. For cancerous conditions, the lead physician would be a gynecologic oncologist. If your gynecologist has diagnosed a malignant condition, he or she will probably refer you to a gynecologic oncologist.

interventional radiologist

A degreed (MD), board certified specialist trained in the diagnostic and therapeutic use of x-rays and radionucleotides, radiation physics and biology, diagnostic ultrasound, and nuclear magnetic resonance imaging.

86. Can my gynecologist tell from first observing my problem whether a hysterectomy will be unavoidable?

Unfortunately, your gynecologist will not be able to tell you immediately whether you should have surgery. All cases require extensive evaluation, which should include a complete medical history, a physical examination, imaging, and laboratory tests. A key question your physician will want answered is whether you have undergone alternate procedures in the past. If so, then the gynecologist will want to know which procedures you have tried.

Just because you have a reproductive-system disorder does not mean that a hysterectomy is inevitable or even necessary. Uterine prolapse, pre-cancerous, and cancerous conditions are exceptions.

87. What if my gynecologist and I have tried numerous alternative treatments? Is undergoing a hysterectomy inevitable?

That depends on several factors that may include: the amount of abnormal bleeding; your degree of pain and discomfort; and your ability to effectively go about your daily routines without some degree of debility. Ultimately, only you can make the decision to have a hysterectomy because you are the one coping with the symptoms. Among the questions you may want to ask yourself is whether the potential benefit of surgery outweighs the risks and costs of the procedure. Additionally, because a hysterectomy also eliminates your ability to have children, you also will have to ask yourself, if you are pre-menopausal, whether you are comfortable with that loss.

88. Given that doctors follow professional guidelines on how to handle certain medical conditions, is it possible for me to read a summary of those guidelines?

Of course you can read the guidelines. The American College of Obstetrics and Gynecology has copies of various treatment guidelines available on its Web site, as do various divisions of the National Institutes of Health (NIH). The NIH sponsors numerous studies about fibroid tumors, endometriosis, and other reproductive health issues, and also carries information on its Web site about treatment, scientific research, and clinical trials. Such patient-oriented information is based on treatment guidelines and other pertinent data that have been gathered about specific conditions.

Guidelines are important because they are derived from evidence-based studies that help determine the best method of treatment for any medical disorder, from a female reproductive condition to virtually any major form of cancer.

The American College of Obstetrics and Gynecology has been proactive in making its guidelines available to the public. A goal of the guidelines is not just to cite the best forms of treatment based on rigorous scientific studies, but also to offer some degree of assurance to patients that medical science has made every possible effort to provide patients with the best of care. Because guidelines are based on clinical studies, usually involving hundreds if not thousands of patients, by reading them you may better understand why doctors almost always tell their patients what they might expect, based on the experience of other patients. Treatment guidelines are continuously updated as new and more conclusive studies are conducted.

But while guidelines are vital to good medical care, they are not recipe books to be followed to the letter in every case. There might be very good reasons why your physician may want to try a certain medication or combination of medications in what is known as an "off label" use. The term *off label* simply means that physicians are free to use an approved medication in a different way, if they believe patients might benefit. You may recall from Question #60 that researchers were testing the breast cancer drug Femara as a treatment for endometriosis. This is an off label use of Femara, a drug that was not approved by the Food and Drug Administration for the treatment of a reproductive disorder. Doctors who had a strong hypothesis that it might help patients with endometriosis first tried Femara in a small clinical study, and the results of that small study paved the way for broader research and a potential new use for the medication.

Getting back to the subject of guidelines, it is important to seek them out and to read them because these are likely the rules that are guiding your care. They are also important in another sense: they will probably help broaden what you know about your own medical condition. Once you have read the treatment guidelines, you are more knowledgeable as a patient and therefore are able to ask your doctor better informed questions about your disorder and accepted methods of treatment.

89. My insurance company says I need a second opinion. Will my gynecologist feel insulted?

Insurance companies are in the business of earning profits. One way to ensure that they do so is to make certain that patients receive effective procedures at the lowest possible cost. Surgeries of all kinds are notoriously expensive and your insurer probably will want you to avoid an operation if at all possible, and that isn't because the company loves you. Insurance companies want to keep the millions of dollars they've charged their customers for premiums. They don't want to spend the cash on expensive medical interventions.

For your own peace of mind, you should actively seek the opinion of another physician to make certain the first doctor's recommendation for surgery is indisputable. Second opinions are important when major surgery is planned, regardless of the reason for the operation. Hysterectomy is just one of many procedures

Second opinions are important when major surgery is planned, regardless of the reason for the operation.

161

for which an insurer may demand a second opinion. In fairness to insurance companies, many are recommending evaluations by a disinterested second party because the companies have found some surgeries and diagnostic tests are performed unnecessarily, and that patients may be better served by a less expensive procedure.

Most insurers will pay for the cost of a second opinion, as will Medicare. In many states, Medicaid also will cover the cost. However, if your insurer is demanding a second opinion but will not cover the expense, you still may consider handling the cost yourself because of the value you will gain by having a second physician review your chart and tests. In instances when an insurer will not pay for the second opinion, it is also possible for you to appeal the refusal. Given that the insurance company demanded the second evaluation, you can make a case to the administrators of your health care insurance plan.

While all of this may seem harassing at a time when you may not be feeling your best physically, bear in mind that a second opinion helps you more than it helps the insurance company. Hysterectomy can have a profound psychological impact on some women. As with any form of surgery, hysterectomy can produce anxiety, but it also causes post-operative pain and may even put you into menopause at an early age. Therefore, you will want to be certain that the procedure is warranted and necessary. You don't want to be misled into an operation that is irreversible.

Finally, you may even want to start a journal that will help you understand where you have been in your journey, and are comfortable with the prospects of having your uterus and possibly other reproductive structures removed, no matter what your age. Keep in mind that a hysterectomy can have a different effect based on how it is performed. For example, if your ovaries are left intact, you will continue to produce your natural flow of hormones. If you are being treated for a condition other than cancer and you have been told that your ovaries should be removed, you certainly will want a second opinion to fully understand the need for the more radical procedure.

Physicians are not insulted when their patients seek second opinions. They are accustomed to their patients going elsewhere for an additional opinion. Your doctor also is well aware that insurers often ask for second opinions and many welcome an evaluation that will likely corroborate his or her medical judgment. Conscientious physicians welcome second opinions and encourage their patients to seek them. Your physician probably has given dozens of second opinions involving the recommendations of other physicians and is familiar with the need to offer an evaluation on another physician's case.

It's easy to say that you have seen your gynecologist for years and fully trust his or her medical judgment, but even in instances where there is a strong bond between doctor and patient, you owe yourself the peace of mind knowing your doctor's diagnosis has been corroborated by another.

Also, it is important to note that standards mandating surgery can differ from one region of the country to another, from one hospital to the next, and even from one physician to another. With that in mind, it again is in your best interest to seek a second opinion. With respect to elective procedures, and a hysterectomy is one of them, you are the final arbiter on whether surgery is best in your case, to determine whether the pain associated with an invasive surgery is worth the time, money, and temporary physical discomfort. The most effective way to make this decision is by listening to what more than one doctor has to say. Every patient who is scheduled to have a hysterectomy or any major surgery should be encouraged by her physician to get a second opinion.

90. Can I seek a second opinion even if my insurance company has not requested one?

Yes, you can seek a second opinion for the same reasons as in Question #89. But this is definitely the type of instance in which an insurer would be least likely to cover the second-opinion cost. Even when the insurer is not making the request, some women want second opinions about a recommendation of hysterectomy. A second opinion can offer peace of mind for the patient for several reasons. A second doctor's evaluation may introduce the patient to a new alternative that her physician may not have offered or did not feel confident performing.

You may recall from Question #48 that in the first few years when uterine artery embolization (UAE) became available, few doctors felt confident performing the procedure, and many others did not refer patients to physicians who were well trained in the technique. Doctors now are finding that UAE is becoming an important option that helps women avoid a hysterectomy.

On the other hand, a second opinion also can confirm that a hysterectomy is the best solution after what may have been a long and frustrating series of alternate treatments that proved futile. As discussed in Question #37, in instances when multiple fibroids have obstructed the uterus growing within its cavity and between its walls, procedures that attempt to remove the fibroids alone may not be possible. When the patient is suffering significant pain and excessive bleeding is causing severe anemia, a hysterectomy may be the best way to achieve relief. The surgery eliminates the source of pain and permanently stops the blood loss.

91. How do I get a second opinion?

Getting a second opinion may require some effort on your part. Your gynecologist can provide a recommendation. But it is probably wise to seek an opinion outside of your physician's own office, especially if your doctor is part of a group practice with other gynecologists. It is likely that they may have discussed your case and share a similar opinion on how it should be handled.

Ideally, it is best to seek a second opinion at a major teaching hospital (which is an institution where medical students, interns, and residents are trained). There you will find expert physicians on staff who would be willing to evaluate your case. Another way of finding a physician is to ask friends or family members, especially women who have had a medical problem similar to your own. If that route is not feasible, you can contact the local medical societies in your area or go online to the Web site of the American College of Obstetrics and Gynecology, which maintains a database of member-

physicians throughout the United States. You may also
elect to ask your family physician to refer you to another
doctor for a second opinion.

92. What if the second opinion differs from the first?

You are an active participant in your health care and
when two doctors render completely different opinions, it is not a time for you to shy away and confess to
being confused. You should ask both physicians how
they reached their conclusions, and why each has such
divergent recommendations. You may also want to
seek a third opinion. A third opinion that corroborates
one of the first two may provide guidance on which
path would be the best for you to take.

93. What medical information do I give the second gynecologist?

All of the medical information that has been gathered
in your case is relevant for a second opinion. That
information includes the following: your medical
records; ultrasound images; medication history; the
outcome of previous alternative procedures; and your
own oral history of your pain, abnormal bleeding, or
both. You can request as many opinions as you wish.
As mentioned in the previous answer, two differing
opinions can seem confusing, leaving the patient
uncertain as to which physician is offering the best
medical judgment in her case. When patients become
their own health advocates, they actively seek answers
to their questions.

When patients become their own health advocates, they actively seek answers to their questions.

PART ELEVEN

When Hysterectomy is Planned: Understanding the Procedure and Your Hospital Stay

Are hysterectomies performed as outpatient procedures or in the hospital? Either way, should I expect to sign a consent form?

How many procedures does the term "hysterectomy" refer to?

Why aren't all hysterectomies performed as vaginal procedures?

More . . .

94. Are hysterectomies performed as outpatient procedures or in the hospital? Either way, should I expect to sign a consent form?

A hysterectomy is major surgery and is performed in the hospital. It is definitely not an outpatient procedure. Usually you are in the hospital for about three days, but your stay may run a day or two longer if you have a chronic medical condition, such as diabetes, high blood pressure, or any other disorder that may require additional vigilance on your doctor's part. A hysterectomy is a frequently performed major operation and rarely do patients experience serious complications. Most medical centers admit patients the morning of surgery, having already performed the necessary blood, urine, and imaging tests on an outpatient basis. In the event that you have not gotten routine pre-surgical tests, your physician will order them once you are admitted to the hospital.

Risks and complications associated with a hysterectomy usually are small but you should be well aware of them before you have the operation. Again, because the operation usually is not an emergency procedure, you should have time to discuss possible risks and complications long before you are admitted to the hospital. Most women who undergo the surgery do not have any complications. For the record, risks can include: possible injury to adjoining structures during the procedure; excessive bleeding; and pulmonary embolus (a blood clot in a lung). Scar tissue can develop in some patients, causing pain and a need for additional surgery to remove adhesions. As with any surgical procedure, there is the possibility of infection as a complication.

Your doctor will inform you of these possibilities before the procedure is performed. Should you develop a fever after your surgery, you should notify your physician immediately because the increase in body temperature could signify infection. Increased pain in the surgical area might be another symptom of infection. Surgical infections have been reduced at most major hospitals around the country due to the administration of antibiotics prior to the operation. Studies have shown that giving patients an antibiotic about a half hour before surgery dramatically lowers the risk of developing a surgical infection. Preventing post-surgical infections relies on your compliance with instructions from your nurse after you are discharged from the hospital. Heeding cautions about sexual activity, bathing (showers are okay) immediately after your hysterectomy, and douching will help reduce the likelihood that you will introduce microorganisms into the surgical area.

All surgeries require an informed consent form; it is the hospital's way of making certain that you have been informed by your physicians about your medical condition and that you understand why you are undergoing surgery. Consent forms are important documents for hospitals because they provide a modicum of legal protection for the institution should a patient later say she was unaware of the type or extent of the surgery she received. Although consent forms differ in wording from one hospital to another, they basically inform you about the operation and its risks.

In addition, the document may inform you that you are permitting the institution's staff to provide medical treatment, which may include, if you are in a teaching hospital, having your case reviewed during rounds by medical students, interns, residents, and other health care providers who are being trained. Interns are recent graduates of medical schools and residents are physicians who are being trained in a medical specialty.

Even though the consent form may state that you are allowing yourself to be treated by providers in training, you have a legal right to change the document, to edit in your preferences, to say that you would prefer not being treated by interns, student nurses, or others who have yet to be licensed. You can do this by having an additional page attached to the document, or you can write your preferences in the margins of the consent form itself. Bear in mind that while you have the right to change the document, you also should have strong reasons for doing so. You should want to make certain that the changes you are adding to the document are in the best interest of your health and recovery.

Along with the consent form that permits the surgery, many institutions have a second document that must be signed, which permits the anesthesiologist to administer medications that will numb pain and put you to sleep during your hysterectomy. As with the document permitting the operation, the second provides legal protection for the hospital, indicating that you have been made aware of the risks associated with anesthesia.

95. How many procedures does the term "hysterectomy" refer to?

The term *hysterectomy* refers to the removal of all or part of the uterus. Here is a list of the various terms and the number of organs involved in the operation. Although your physician may or may not use such specific medical terminology, these are some terms you will want to know.

Abdominal Procedures

- TAH (Total Abdominal Hysterectomy): This surgical procedure refers to the removal of the uterus and the cervix.
- TAH-BSO (Total Abdominal Hysterectomy with Bilateral Salpingo-Oophorectomy): In this surgical procedure, the uterus, cervix, both fallopian tubes, and both ovaries are removed.
- TAH-RSO (Total Abdominal Hysterectomy with Right Salpingo-Oophorectomy): A surgical procedure where the uterus, cervix, right fallopian tube, and right ovary are removed.
- TAH-LSO (Total Abdominal Hysterectomy with Left Salpingo-Oophorectomy): A surgical procedure where the uterus, cervix, left fallopian tube, and left ovary are removed.
- Supracervical Abdominal Hysterectomy: The uterus is removed and the cervix is left intact.

Vaginal Procedures

- TVH (Total Vaginal Hysterectomy): A surgery performed through the vagina to remove the uterus.
- TVH-BSO (Total Vaginal Hysterectomy with Bilateral Salpingo-Oophorectomy): A surgery performed through the vagina to remove the uterus, fallopian tubes, and both ovaries; also referred to as a total or complete hysterectomy.
- LAVH (Laparoscopic Vaginal Hysterectomy): A minimally invasive procedure using a laparoscope to visualize the pelvic region and to aid in the removal of the uterus through the vagina.

96. How does my doctor know which procedure is right for me, and why does the procedure my doctor recommends have an impact on recuperation?

As mentioned in Question #7, a hysterectomy can be performed either abdominally or vaginally. Even though a significant percentage of the procedures in the United States are still performed as abdominal procedures, numerous studies have shown that vaginal hysterectomies are the procedure of choice for non-malignant conditions. Research has demonstrated that vaginal procedures are less invasive, produce less post-operative pain, require less time for recuperation, and are generally less costly. Compared with abdominal hysterectomies there is less contact and manipulation of the large intestine and a significantly lower possibility of post-operative infection.

The potential for infection is lower with a vaginal procedure because the surgery is less invasive. This is a plus for patients because it also means less time on antibiotics after surgery. For a majority of women undergoing vaginal procedures, bowel function returns sooner after this form of hysterectomy, discharge from the hospital is sooner, and recuperation time at home is shorter. Additionally, patients prefer a vaginal procedure because there is no scar to contend with afterward.

Finally, the more invasive any surgical procedure, the longer it will take for you to recover. Your recovery roughly relates to the extensiveness of your surgery, and this is not strictly a matter concerning those structures that are removed in a hysterectomy. During the operation, not only are certain organs, structures, or glands removed, others that remain get jostled during surgery. This is especially true for those who undergo an abdominal procedure during which organs and structures that are not being removed get moved around a bit as the surgeon removes the uterus. Keep in mind that the area in which the surgery is being conducted is very small, so it takes these structures a little time to settle into place and for your body to resume its normal function after surgery.

97. Why aren't all hysterectomies performed as vaginal procedures?

Individual medical circumstances govern how a hysterectomy should be performed. The choice to perform the surgery through an abdominal or vaginal incision, therefore, is based on your specific circumstances. If, for example, you are being treated for endometriosis in which numerous adhesions throughout the abdominal tract have affected your reproductive organs and intestines, it is not likely that your physician will recommend a vaginal procedure. The same is true if you are being treated for a reproductive tract cancer, for you an abdominal surgery will be the procedure of choice.

If you have very large fibroids, a condition that used to be a textbook reason for an abdominal hysterectomy, it is likely that such an operation can be performed vaginally because of advances in surgical techniques. No matter which method is being recommended, you should thoroughly discuss your operation with your physician weeks before you are scheduled to undergo the procedure, and make certain that your physician understands your preference and explains how your choice can or cannot be accommodated.

Hysterectomies rarely are performed as emergency procedures. This means that there is sufficient time for you to have such a discussion with your doctor so that you are fully aware of what will happen in the surgical suite. If for any reason you are in disagreement with your physician, who may suggest an abdominal operation when you may prefer a vaginal one, you are free to seek a second opinion, just as you might have done to determine whether the surgery was warranted in the first place.

PART TWELVE

Life After a Hysterectomy

Should I still be on birth control pills or
some other method of birth control?

Should I expect to be incontinent
after a hysterectomy?

What can I expect during my recovery and beyond?
Will I gain weight?

More . . .

98. I recently had a hysterectomy and my doctor removed my left fallopian tube and ovary. Should I still be on birth control pills or some other method of birth control? My sex life is as active now as it was before surgery.

We have explained throughout this book that a hysterectomy is the removal of the uterus. Without a uterus, you are forever prevented from becoming pregnant or having menstrual periods. Your menstrual periods cease because there is no uterine lining to shed monthly. If you were told that your surgery was a hysterectomy and if your physician also told you that you would no longer have the capacity to become pregnant, then you should accept the fact that your reproductive days are over.

For the record, there have been a few documented cases of tubal pregnancies following a hysterectomy, but it cannot be stressed more emphatically that such cases are extraordinarily rare. Most instances of post-hysterectomy ectopic pregnancies (any pregnancy occurring outside the uterus) occur shortly after a hysterectomy and are found in a remaining fallopian tube. Doctors who have reported post-hysterectomy tubal pregnancies in medical journals have made note of their extreme rarity and generally agree the pregnancies resulted from a fertilized egg that was coincidentally in a fallopian tube at the time of surgery.

None of these pregnancies were sustainable and never could have been carried to term because they pose a life-threatening risk of tubal rupture and internal bleeding. Moreover, without a uterus, the gateway to the tubes is no longer present. This prevents any entrance by sperm, which explains why hysterectomy is viewed as the most effective method of sterilization.

Without a uterus, there is no place for a placenta to implant or for the fetus to be properly nourished. Among the post-hysterectomy cases of pregnancy that have been reported worldwide, virtually all were treated as emergencies when women were rushed into hospitals complaining of extreme abdominal pain. With the advent of Internet blogs and boards, women increasingly have been reporting post-hysterectomy symptoms of pregnancy. Themes appearing often in many of the threads are of specific pregnancy-like symptoms such as breast tenderness and lower abdominal flutters that have been reported as feeling similar to fetal activity.

Some women say they've noticed an enlargement of their abdomens to about the size of a five-month pregnancy. In response to these reports, some bloggers have written that they have had their symptoms checked by doctors. The physicians, in turn, ordered ultrasound examinations and pregnancy tests. But the symptoms turned out to be false alarms. It really makes you wonder if the doctors were uncertain what kind of surgery they had performed.

Psychologists emphasize that the loss of reproductive capability can affect some women very profoundly. When the ovaries are left intact after hysterectomy in pre-menopausal women, the body is still responding to the same hormones. It is likely that without the pain or excessive bleeding associated with fibroids, or endometriosis or adenomyosis, or whatever led to a hysterectomy, some women are more acutely aware of symptoms associated with cycling hormones. Symptoms such as breast tenderness may be mistaken as a sign of early pregnancy. But while phantom pregnancies seem to be a growing topic on the Internet, genuine post-hysterectomy pregnancy is an incredibly rare and life-threatening event.

Genuine post-hysterectomy pregnancy is an incredibly rare and life-threatening event.

99. Should I expect to be incontinent after a hysterectomy?

You should not experience incontinence (inability to prevent leakage of urine or feces) after your hysterectomy. This is not to say that urinary incontinence is not a concern. It increasingly has become a concern among medical researchers as they have begun to investigate subtler symptoms that may not occur immediately, but could take years to manifest.

A study sponsored by the Agency for Healthcare Research suggested that women affected by moderate-to-severe urinary incontinence prior to their hysterectomies seemed to improve for at least two years after their operations. Nevertheless, the same investigation revealed that women with mild incontinence or no history of the condition had a 10% risk of either worsening symptoms or development of the disorder.

More provocative are studies that have tried to determine who the most vulnerable type might be and when urinary incontinence is most likely to occur. One major study found incontinence not manifest for 20 to 30 years after a hysterectomy, a possibility that, on first blush, seems incomprehensible until put into the perspective of those medical researchers who are looking into the matter. They correlate the slow onset of urinary incontinence to the similarly slow onset of incontinence that sometimes follows childbirth. Some women experience pelvic nerve damage during childbirth, which years later can lead to urinary incontinence. The same, they say, may be true for a certain percentage of women after hysterectomy.

One of the leading scientific papers to draw an association between hysterectomy and urinary incontinence was authored by researchers at the University of California, San Francisco, who published their results in the British medical journal *The Lancet*. They postulate that urinary incontinence occurring as a possible long-term consequence of hysterectomy can take up to three decades to emerge. Childbirth-induced incontinence, the San Francisco team reported, can have a delay of five to ten years. Whether incontinence is associated with hysterectomy or with childbirth, the result can be a chronic inability to hold urine without leakage, a situation that can create a serious quality of life concern.

In the *Lancet* study, the UCSF researchers, led by Dr. Jeannette S. Brown, professor of obstetrics and gynecology, divided cases by age and a host of other variables. Dr. Brown and her colleagues concluded that urinary incontinence was 40% more likely in women who had undergone a hysterectomy than for women who had not had the surgery. Narrowing their data further to look at specific age groups, Dr. Brown and her team found that the likelihood of developing incontinence was 60% more likely in women past age 60 than for those who were younger. The researchers did not investigate which type of incontinence occurred most frequently, that is, whether it was urge, stress, or mixed incontinence.

Incontinence is a major health concern in the United States, affecting about 13 million people. This particular *Lancet* study is known as a meta-analysis, which means that several major studies on the subject were pooled and re-analyzed to reach a conclusion. As with any meta-analysis, the findings essentially generate a hypothesis, which in this case states that hysterectomy may lead to urinary incontinence in some older women. With the hypothesis now in hand, the scientific community essentially has been challenged to conduct more rigorous studies to prove or disprove the hypothesis. Anecdotal evidence (non-scientifically studied reports from individuals) suggests that there may be a link between the surgery and incontinence in some women.

100. What can I expect during my recovery and beyond? Will I gain weight?

There is no one-size-fits-all scenario involving recovery from hysterectomy. Some women bounce back sooner than others, saying they felt like themselves a lot faster than they initially thought. But no matter how they describe it, no one goes through the recovery period in a few days. Most women point to a gradual return to their personal level of normalcy, some resuming their old routines sooner than others. Bear in mind that it takes time for abdominal organs to reposition, especially if you have undergone an abdominal operation. Your body will take time to resume its normal bowel activity. If you had an abdominal surgery, you will need time for the surgical site to heal. You will probably feel fatigued. Some women remark that they're surprised by how tired they felt after their operation. Resuming a rigorous exercise regimen may have to wait for several weeks while you heal physically and emotionally. Hysterectomy, whether you welcome the relief it brings after years of abnormal bleeding, does represent a loss. Some women grieve, and that takes time.

Another major issue immediately following surgery and for a while afterward, for some women, is pain. Post-operative pain is to be expected but, as mentioned elsewhere in the text, the type of operation your doctor performed will largely influence the degree of pain you feel afterward. You may recall that abdominal surgeries produce more pain and underlie a longer recovery period than vaginal hysterectomies. You will be treated for pain while in the hospital and your physician will recommend pain medication upon discharge. Post-operative pain can range from mild to severe and can last from days to weeks. If a nerve is injured during the surgery, which is a rare event, then the pain after a hysterectomy might last for years.

Increasingly, some doctors have begun treating women with a device called a "pain relief ball," which has been used following a number of different gynecologic surgeries, including C-sections. Actually, the so-called ball is a balloon-like mechanism that releases medication into the surgical site. The drug is non-narcotic, which means that you can avoid any side effects associated with those medications.

For mild pain, there is a wide range of options. Your physician might recommend one of the old medicine cabinet standbys: acetaminophen (sold as Tylenol) or any of the widely prescribed non-steroidal anti-inflammatory drugs (NSAIDs), which includes naproxen, ibuprofen, and enteric-coated aspirin, among others. Your health care provider will try to match the medication to the level of pain you are experiencing. Sometimes this is done by asking you to gauge on a scale of 1 to 10, with 10 being worst, where you would pinpoint your level of discomfort.

Glossary

Abdominal surgeries: Type of surgical procedure performed through an incision similar to the kind made for a Caesarean section.

Abnormal uterine bleeding: A disorder caused by any one of several underlying reproductive system conditions; characterized by excessive bleeding and/or blood clots that may lead to anemia.

Adenomyosis: A very painful condition characterized by the infiltration of glandular tissue from the lining of the uterus into the muscular portion of the uterine walls.

Adhesions: Fibrous bands of tissue that abnormally cling to nearby structures; may cause major structures (e.g., ovary, outer walls of the uterus and bladder) to become stuck together. The condition produces extraordinary pain.

Anemia: A disorder in which there is a low red blood cell count; red blood cells carry less oxygen. Anemia can result in fatigue and exhaustion. If untreated may prove life-threatening.

Anovulatory: Menstrual periods in which an egg is not produced.

Atypia: A term pathologists use to describe abnormal cells.

Bilateral oophorectomy: Surgical removal of both ovaries.

Bimanual examination: A type of investigation used for diagnosis, where the physician places two lubricated gloved fingers into the vagina and pushes upward while at the same time, on the outside of the lower abdomen, presses down with the other hand; this action allows your gynecologist to feel any growths in the uterus or on the ovaries.

Biopsy: A surgical procedure in which a tiny sample of tissue is removed so that the cells can be viewed under a microscope and analyzed.

Birth control medications: Hormone-based drugs used primarily to prevent conception. Also used as treatments for fibroids and other reproductive system disorders.

Cancer: Any malignant development caused by abnormal and uncontrolled growth of cells. Some cancers grow rapidly and invade surrounding tissues and organs; others are more indolent and grow slowly.

Cervical dysplasia: The abnormal growth of cells on the surface of the cervix (which is the entrance to the uterus).

Cervical intraepithelial neoplasia (CIN): A pre-cancerous condition caused by an abnormal growth of cells on the surface of the cervix. These cells can linger for long periods in a pre-cancerous state before advancing to invasive cancer.

Cervical polyps: Tiny growths that protrude inside the uterus and may be a source of abnormal bleeding.

Cervix: The neck at the lower end of the uterus. It connects the uterus to the vagina. The cervix dilates during labor to allow the birth of a baby.

Complex hyperplasia: A term used by pathologists to define an overgrowth of cells in the uterus where the proliferation is so excessive that the structure of the uterus itself has changed. Microscopically, the infinitesimal glands of the endometrium can be seen crowding one another. The endometrium's stroma cells also exhibit marked proliferation.

Cryomyolysis: A surgical method that involves freezing fibroids, which forces them to shrink.

Depression: A mental condition marked by sadness, inactivity, and an inability to think clearly. Depression is also characterized by feelings of dejection or hopelessness, and a significant increase or decrease in sleeping. In severe cases there may be suicidal tendencies.

Dermatopontin: A protein made by the body to prevent cells from straying into aberrant patterns of growth. Researchers have associated low levels of the protein with the development of fibroid tumors.

Dilation and curettage (D&C): A diagnostic procedure performed when the woman is under general anesthesia or an epidural; the cervix is dilated, and then with a spoon-shaped instrument called a curette, the uterus is scraped. The resulting tissue specimen is sent to a laboratory for analysis.

Dysfunctional uterine bleeding (DUB): Excessive uterine bleeding.

Endometrial cancer: A malignancy that affects cells lining the uterus.

Endometrial hyperplasia: A condition where there is thickening of the uterine lining (overgrowth of cells in the endometrium) that may cause excessive bleeding.

Endometrial polyps: Small benign growths that protrude into the uterus.

Endometrium: The inner lining of the uterus.

Endometrial ablation: An outpatient procedure that may involve a laser (or other source) to eliminate the cells lining the uterus. The procedure may make conception impossible.

Endometriosis: A reproductive system disorder where tissue from the inner lining of the uterus grows in places it should not be. Endometrial tissue can implant itself anywhere in the pelvic area (including the ovaries, the bladder, and even the large intestine), leading to scar tissue and pain during sexual intercourse and bowel movements. Some patients report a constant dull pain in the abdomen, and an escalation in the degree of pain during menstruation.

Epidural: A procedure in which nerves are numbed from the waist down.

Estrogen: A hormone formed by the ovaries, the placenta during pregnancy, and, to a lesser extent, by fat cells with the aid of an enzyme called aromatase. Estrogen stimulates secondary sex characteristics, such as the growth of breasts, and exerts systemic effects (i.e., growth and maturation of long bones, and control of the menstrual cycle).

Fallopian tubes: Also known as the oviducts; located at the top part of the uterus (the fundus), they are the conduits through which eggs cells (ova) are transported to the uterus. At their uppermost ends, the tubes have fingerlike projections that sweep eggs from the ovaries. Each tube measures about four inches in length and possesses contractile capability, a motion that allows them to propel an egg into the uterus.

Follicle cells: A type of cell located in the ovary that produces eggs.

Follicle-stimulating hormone (FSH): Produced by the pituitary gland in the brain; when suppressed by estrogen, FSH inhibits ovulation in the earlier phase of the menstrual cycle.

Gonadotrophin-releasing hormone agonists (GnRHa): A group of medications that prevent the body from making estrogen and progesterone. These medications can be prescribed to help to reduce the size of fibroid tumors by creating a pseudo-state of menopause.

Gynecologist: A medical doctor (MD) who has completed a residency specializing in disorders of the female reproductive tract as well as issues involving endocrinology and reproductive physiology.

Gynecologic oncologist: A gynecologist who has completed a post-residency fellowship in diagnosing and treating cancer of the female reproductive organs.

Hereditary predisposition: Suggests the likelihood that a medical condition has a familial link.

Hormone replacement therapy (HRT): Medication containing one or more female hormones. Most often HRT is used to treat symptoms of menopause (hot flashes, vaginal dryness, mood swings, sleep disorders, and decreased sexual desire). Estrogen replacement therapy is a form of HRT that includes only the estrogen hormone.

Hysterectomy: The surgical removal of the uterus (the womb).

Hysteroscopy: A diagnostic procedure that uses a telescopic instrument to inspect the uterus.

Immune system dysfunction: A theory of endometriosis which suggests the disorder results from the immune system's failure to destroy any endometrial cells remaining after menstruation.

Informed consent form: A legal document that explains any invasive medical procedure, which must be read and signed by the patient in advance. Most forms describe the procedure and indicate that you have been informed of its risks and benefits.

Interligamentous fibroid: A type of growth that develops within a ligament that supports the uterus in the pelvic area.

Interventional radiologist: A medical doctor (MD) who has completed a residency in radiology as well as post-residency training in Interventional radiology

Intramural fibroid: A type of fibroid that grows between the smooth muscular walls of the uterus; may cause symptoms similar to submucosal and subserosal fibroids.

Laparoscope: A very small, thin surgical instrument that allows inspection of the abdominal organs through a tiny camera attached to the device.

Laser: A high-energy light source that emits a beam in a specified wavelength. A laser can quickly vaporize abnormalities with its heat.

Menorrhagia: Heavy menstrual bleeding within a normal cycle; may be a symptom of dysfunctional uterine bleeding.

Menstruation: A discharge of blood, secretions, and tissue fragments from the uterus at regular intervals, usually after ovulation.

Metaplasia: A theory of endometriosis suggesting that endometrial islands are deposited outside of the uterus before birth, during the earliest phases of fetal development. As an adult, these deposits attempt to function as if they, too, are a uterus.

Metrorrhagia: Bleeding between menstrual periods; may be a symptom of dysfunctional uterine bleeding.

Mifepristone: A synthetic steroid hormone that blocks the action of progesterone; used in a few small studies of women with fibroids; capable of slowing or sometimes stopping fibroid growth.

Myolysis: A surgical procedure in which the blood supply to fibroids is halted, causing fibroids to shrink and die.

Myomectomy: A type of surgery to remove an individual fibroid.

Nonsteroidal anti-inflammatory drugs (NSAIDs): A group of medications (aspirin, ibuprofen, and naproxen) that reduce inflammation and simultaneously affect the natural hormone-like fatty acids known as prostaglandins, which are a major source of pain and inflammation.

Oophorectomy: Removal of the ovaries; can trigger the immediate onset of menopause and menopausal symptoms, including: hot flashes, night sweats, mood swings, vaginal dryness, and short-term memory loss.

Osteopenia: A condition of decreased calcification or density of bone.

Ovary: Twin oval-shaped glands about the size of an almond; located on either side of the uterus that contain thousands of ova (also known as germ cells). One egg is released per month, starting at puberty and continuing in a clocklike pattern throughout most of the reproductive years.

Parasitic fibroid: A growth that develops outside of the uterus, such as on the pelvic wall.

Pedunculated fibroids: A type of fibroid that grows on a stalk usually on the outside of the uterus.

Pelvic congestion syndrome: A type of disorder where the veins that nourish the uterus widen, thus causing blood to pool and resulting in debilitating pain.

Pelvic inflammatory disease (PID): Acute or chronic inflammation of female pelvic structures (endometrium, uterine tubes, pelvic peritoneum) due to infection (gonorrhea, chlamydia, and other organisms). If untreated, PID can result in scarring and infertility.

Pelvic pressure: A sensation of "fullness" in the abdomen; can be caused by fibroids.

Perimenopause: A stage in a woman's life when the ovaries no longer function as in youth; precursor of menopause.

Pessary: A plastic device that, when placed in the vagina, helps to support the uterus.

Polymenorrhea: Menstrual periods that occur far too frequently, usually within a cycle of less than 21 days; may be a symptom of dysfunctional uterine bleeding.

Progesterone: A sex hormone that prepares the uterus for pregnancy.

Prostaglandins: A family of potent hormone-like fatty acids secreted by an array of tissues that can serve as a source of pain and inflammation. Prostaglandins have been implicated in a wide variety of pain syndromes from migraine headaches to uterine cramps.

Rectovaginal examination: A type of investigation used for diagnosis, where the physician simultaneously places one lubricated gloved finger in the vagina and another in the rectum; important test for pelvic abnormalities.

Retrograde menstruation: A theory that endometriosis is a process of reverse menstruation where, instead of flowing out of the body, the blood backs up into the reproductive system, moving into the fallopian tubes and elsewhere throughout the pelvic region. Instead of being discarded as menstrual waste, this residue from the uterus deposits itself throughout the pelvic area and continues to bleed and function as if it were still lining the uterus.

Sarcoma: A highly malignant type of tumor; connective tissue neoplasm.

Simple hyperplasia: A condition typified by an overgrowth of cells in the uterus; the inner lining of the uterus becomes thickened. Despite such cellular proliferation, the uterine structure remains unchanged and there is no evidence of atypical or pre-cancerous cells. Also called mild, Swiss cheese, and cystic.

Simple endometrial hyperplasia with atypia: A term used by pathologists for cells that demonstrate an abnormality and possess about an 8% chance of becoming cancerous. The usual recommendation for patients is a D&C, progestin therapy, and periodic monitoring.

Submucous or submucosal fibroid: A type of fibroid tumor that develops directly beneath the surface of the endometrium. The large number of blood vessels on its surface can bleed and trigger pain. These fibroids tend to prevent the uterine muscle's ability to properly contract because they distort the shape and function of the organ; they can grow to a size that obstructs the fallopian tubes and also may distort the uterine lining as they grow, causing menstrual irregularities. They may even become pedunculated and project into the cervix or even the vagina.

Subtotal hysterectomy: The surgical removal of the pear-shaped uterus, leaving the cervix in place.

Total abdominal hysterectomy with bilateral salpingo-oophorectomy (TAH-BSO): A type of hysterectomy that involves the removal of the uterus, the fallopian tubes, and both ovaries.

Total hysterectomy: The surgical removal of the uterus and cervix.

Ultrasound: A type of imaging machine that uses high frequency soundwaves for medical diagnoses.

Uterine artery embolization: A surgical technique that blocks the blood supply to problematic fibroids.

Uterine fibroids: Benign tumors that can cause severe abnormal bleeding and extreme pain; also known as fibromyoma, leiomyoma, and myoma. May trigger heavy menstrual bleeding, disabling cramps, unpredictable bleeding between periods, and may underlie serious anemia and exhaustion.

Uterine prolapse: Also known as pelvic relaxation, this condition occurs when the ligaments that hold the uterus and/or bladder in place loosen. Severe weakening may allow the organ(s) to protrude through the vagina.

Urinary incontinenc1e: An inability to prevent the excretion of urine.

Uterus: Also called the womb; a pear-shaped hollow organ about three inches long and two inches wide at its top; has a role in the monthly menstrual cycle, provides an environment for the growth and nourishment of a developing fetus, and produces mild contractile waves as part of the female sexual response.

Vagina: The passageway from the outside of the body to the reproductive system's interior.

Vaginal hysterectomy: Type of surgery that removes the uterus through the vagina.

Vascular and/or lymphatic transport: A theory of endometriosis where endometrial implants are carried to inappropriate sites in the body via the bloodstream, the lymphatic system, or both.

Appendix

Organizations

American College of Obstetricians and Gynecologists
www.acog.org
By Telephone: (202) 638-5577
By Mail: 409 12th Street SW, Washington, DC 20090-6920

American College of Surgeons
www.facs.org
By Telephone: (312) 202-5000
Toll Free: 1-800-621-4111
By Mail: 633 North Saint Clair Street, Chicago, IL 60611-3211

American Chronic Pain Association
www.theacpa.org
By Telephone: 1-800-533-3231
By Mail: P.O. Box 850, Rocklin, CA 95677

American Pain Society
www.ampainsoc.org
By Telephone: (847) 375-4715
By Mail: 4700 West Lake Avenue, Glenview, IL 60025

American Social Health Association
www.ashastd.org
By Telephone: (919) 361-8400
By Mail: P.O. Box 13827, Research Triangle Park, NC 27709

Centers for Disease Control and Prevention
www.cdc.gov
By Telephone: (404) 639-3534
Toll Free: 1-800-311-3435
By Mail: U.S. Centers for Disease Control and Prevention, 1600 Clifton Road, Atlanta, GA 30333

Center for Uterine Fibroids
www.fibroids.net
The Center is in Boston at Brigham and Women's Hospital, an affiliate of Harvard Medical School. Researchers conduct genetic studies on the causes of uterine fibroids. Information is maintained on website about fibroids and various forms of treatment.
By Telephone: 1-800-722-5520 (ask operator for 525-4434)
By Mail: 77 Avenue Louis Pasteur, 160 New Research Building, Boston, MA 02115

Endometriosis Association (Endo-Online)
www.endometriosisassn.org
By Telephone: (414) 355-2200
By Mail: 8585 North 76th Place, Milwaukee, WI 53223

Endometriosis Research Center, World Headquarters
www.endocenter.org
By Telephone: (561) 274-7442
Toll Free: 1-800-239-7289
By Mail: 630 Ibis Drive, Delray Beach, FL 33444

Fibroids1.com
www.fibroids1.com
By Telephone: (617) 576-9400
By Mail: 222 Third Street, Cambridge, MA 02142

Fibroid Treatment Collective
www.fibroids.com
This Web site contains information about uterine embolization.
By Telephone: (310) 208-2442
Toll Free: 1-866-362-6463
By Mail: 100 UCLA Medical Plaza, Suite 310, Los Angeles, CA 90095-96211

Health Insurance Association of America
www.hiaa.org
By Telephone: 202-824-1600
By Mail: 555 13th Street NW, Suite 600, Washington, DC 20004-1109

Health Resources and Services Administration
Hill Burton Program (for information about free or low-cost health-care offered in some areas)
www.hrsa.gov/osp/dfcr/about/aboutdiv.htm
By Telephone: (301) 443-5656
Toll Free: 1-800-638-0742/1-800-492-0359 (if calling from Maryland)
By Mail: Health Resources and Services Administration, U.S. Department of Health and Human Services, Parklawn Building, 5600 Fishers Lane, Rockville, MD 20857

HERS Foundation
Hysterectomy Alternatives and Aftereffects
www.hersfoundation.org
By Telephone: (610) 667-7757
Toll Free: 1-888-750-HERS or 1-888-750-4377
By Mail: 422 Bryn Mawr Avenue, Bala Cynwyd, PA 19004

Hysterectomy Resource Center
www.obgyn.net/hysterectomy-resource-center
By Telephone: (763) 416-3000
Toll Free: 1-866-724-3101
By Mail: Gyrus Medical, 6655 Wedgwood Road, Suite 160, Maple Grove, MN 55311

HysterSisters, Inc.
www.hystersisters.com
By Telephone: (940) 898-0070
By Mail: 700 Londonderry Lane, Denton, TX 76205

Institute for Female Alternative Medicine
www.alternativesurgery.com/education/hysterectomy.php
The Institute's Web site has information about adenomyosis,
endometriosis, fibroids, ovarian cysts, hysterectomy, etc.
By Telephone: 1-800-505-4326
By Mail: 1500 Central Avenue, Glendale, CA 91204

National Uterine Fibroids Foundation
www.nuff.org
By Telephone: (719) 633-3454
By Mail: P.O. Box 9688, Colorado Springs, CO 80932-0688

National Women's Health Network
www.womenshealthnetwork.org
By Telephone: (202) 628-7814
By Mail: 514 10th Street, Washington, DC 20004

National Women's Health Resource Center
www.healthywomen.org
By Telephone: 1-877-986-9472
By Mail: 157 Broad Street, Suite 315, Red Bank, NJ 07701

RESOLVE: The National Infertility Association
www.resolve.org
By Telephone: (301) 652-9375
By Mail: 7910 Woodmont Avenue, Suite 1350, Bethesda, MD
20814

Web Page Resources

Alternatives to Hysterectomy
www.althysterectomy.org

Avoiding Hysterectomy
www.nohysterectomy.com

Endometriosis Information
Various Internet-based organizations offer information about endometriosis:

1. www.endofacts.com (from the maker of Lupon Depot)
2. www.endometriosis.org
3. www.endozone.org
4. www.emedicinehealth.com/endometriosis
5. www.topix.net/health/endometriosis

Endometriosis During Teen Years
www.youngwomenshealth.org/endoinfo.html

Fibroids
1. www.fibroidfacts.com (from the maker of Lupron Depot)
2. www.nlm.nih.gov/medlineplus/ency/article/000914.htm (from Medline Plus, a service of the National Library of Medicine and the National Institutes of Health)
3. www.fda.gov/womens/getthefacts/fibroids.html (Food and Drug Administration Fact Sheet on Fibroids)
4. www.mayoclinic.com/health/uterine-fibroids/UF99999 (guide on fibroids from the renowned Mayo Clinic)
5. www.womenshealthmatters.ca/centres/pelvic_health/fibroids (information from the New Women's College Hospital in Ontario, Canada)

Hysterectomy Information
www.4woman.gov/faq/hysterectomy.htm
www.hysterectomy.net (sponsored by HysterSisters.com)
www.yoursurgery.com

Women's Health Issues
Agency for Healthcare Research and Quality
www.ahrq.gov/consumer

Cancer

American Cancer Society
www.cancer.org
By Telephone: 1-800-ACS-2345
By Mail: American Cancer Society National Home Office, 1599
Clifton Road, Atlanta, GA 30329

Gynecologic Cancer Foundation
www.wcn.org
By Telephone: (312) 644-6610
By Mail: 230 West Monroe, Suite 2528, Chicago, IL 60606-4267

National Cancer Institute
www.cancer.gov/cancertopics/types/cervical
www.cancer.gove/cancertopics/types/endometrial
www.cancer,gov/cancertopics/types/ovarian
By Telephone: (301) 435-3848 (Public Information)
By Mail: National Cancer Institute Public Information Office
Building 31, Room 10A31, 31 Center Drive, MSC 2580,
Bethesda, MD 20892

National Cervical Cancer Coalition
www.nccc-online.org
By Telephone: (818) 685-5531
By Mail: 7247 Hayvenhurst Avenue, Suite A-7, Van Nuys, CA 91406

National Comprehensive Cancer Network
www.nccn.org
By Telephone: 1-888-909-6226
By Mail: 50 Huntingdon Pike, Suite 200, Rockledge PA 19046

Ovarian Cancer National Alliance
www.ovariancancer.org
By Telephone: (202) 331-1332
By Mail: 910 17th Street, NW Washington, DC 20006

Society of Gynecologic Oncologists
A professional organization for physicians who treat gynecologic cancers; the Web site has information for patients.
www.sgo.org
By Telephone: (312) 235-4060
By Mail: 230 West Monroe, Suite 710, Chicago, IL 6060

Finding a Doctor

Find an Ob-Gyn (*American College of Obstetricians and Gynecologists*)
www.acog.org/member-lookup/disclaimer.cfm
The database allows patients to search for a gynecologist who is a member of the American College of Obstetricians and Gynecologists by name or zip code.

AIM DocFinder (*State Medical Board Executive Directors*)
www.docboard.org
Nonprofit organization providing a health professional licensing database

AMA Physician Select (*American Medical Association*)
www.ama-assn.org/aps/amahg.htm
AMA database of demographic and professional information on individual physicians throughout the United States

Verifying credentials (*American Board of Medical Specialties*)
www.abms.org
Provides verification of physician qualifications and has lists of
specialists

Finding a Hospital

Hospital Select
www.hospitalselect.com/curb_db/owa/sp_hospselect.main
Database searchable by a hospital's name, city, state or zip code.
Information includes basic data, such as number of beds, utilization
and accreditation.

Best Hospitals Finder (*U.S. News & World Report*)
www.usnews.com/usnews/nycu/health/hosptl/tophosp.htm
The *U.S. News & World Report* hospital rankings are designed to
assist patients in their searchfor the highest level of medical care.
Database is searchable by specialty.

Best HMOs Finder (*U.S. News & World Report*)
www.usnews.com/usnews/nycu/health/hetophmo.htm
U.S. News & World Report guide to choosing a managed care
option

Index

E

ectopic pregnancies, 58
  caused by PID, 138
  post-hysterectomy, 176
egg production, 34, 59. *See also* fallopian tubes
  fibroid obstruction, 76, 78
  perimenopause and, 65
embolization, 99
emergency hysterectomies, 174
emotional impact, 177–178
  of chronic bleeding, 39
  fibroids, 77
  of hysterectomy, 42–44
endometrial ablation, 38, 128, 184
endometrial cancer, 52–53, 149–152, 184
endometrial hyperplasia, 38, 145–148, 184
endometrial polyps, 50, 184
endometriosis, 4, 104–124
  cancer and, 120–121.
    See also endometrial cancer
  cause of, 107–109
  defined, 104, 185
  estrogen as cause, 62
  fertility problems, 107, 110, 111, 118–120
  lifestyle choices, 121–122
  nonsurgical treatment for, 112–115
  pain relief, 39–41
  restoring fertility after treatment, 123–124
  surgery other than hysterectomy, 115–117
  symptoms and diagnosis, 109–111
  Web page resources, 195
endometriosis interna. *See* adenomyosis
endometrium, 38, 56, 184
environmental causes of fibroids, 74
epidural, defined, 185
estradiol, 62
estrogen, 59, 60, 62–63
  defined, 185
  egg production and, 36
  endometrial cancer, 151
  endometrial hyperplasia, 146–147
  endometriosis, 105
  growth of uterine fibroids, 72, 74
  menstrual cycle and, 50
  pelvic congestion syndrome, 130
  replacement of, 6. *See also* hormone replacement therapy
  synthetic, 61
ethnicity, fibroid development and, 81–82

excessive or persistent bleeding.
    See abnormal uterine bleeding
exercise
  endometriosis and, 121–122
  fibroids and, 85
  following surgery, 180–181

F

fallopian tubes, 58
  defined, 185
  endometrial deposits on.
    See endometriosis
  infection of. *See* PID (pelvic inflammatory disease)
  obstructed with fibroids, 76, 78
  tubal (ectopic) pregnancies, 58, 138, 176
family, hysterectomies among, 51
fatigue, 32–39, 48
  following surgery, 180–181
fear. *See* stress
fecal incontinence. *See* incontinence
female reproductive system, healthy, 56–65
Femara (letrozole), 118–120, 160
fertility. *See* childbearing
fibroid tumors. *See* uterine fibroids
fibroids
  childbearing and miscarriage, 77–79
  important facts about, 87–88
  lifestyle and body weight, 84–86
  as reason for hysterectomy, 86–87
  surgical treatment for, 94–101.
    See also myolysis; myomectomy; uterine artery embolization
  testing for, 79–80
  therapeutic treatment and pain relief, 88–94
  Web page resources, 195–196
  when and how they develop, 80–84, 87
fibromyoma. *See* uterine fibroids
finding a doctor or hospital, 197–198
fish oil capsules for endometriosis, 122
follicle cells, 36, 185
follicle-stimulating hormone (FSH), 60–61, 185
future of hysterectomy, 11

G

genetic predisposition
  defined, 185
  endometriosis, 105, 108
  family members who had hysterectomies, 186
  uterine fibroids, 74